A Physicians's

Guide To Natural

Health Products

That Work

1

For information regarding rights or permissions, please contact:

Dr. James A. Howenstine, 7333 N.W. 54th St. Miami, Florida, 33166

ISBN 0-9705684-8-7

Library of Congress Card Number: 2001094553

Published by Penhurst Books
Miami, Florida

Penhurst Books

Cover Design by Bob Wagner Designs

Printed in the United States of America

Dedication

This book is dedicated to all who are searching for better health. And God said "See, I have given you every herb that yields seed which is on the face of all the earth, and every tree whose fruit yields seed; to you it shall be for food." Genesis 1:29

5 Basic Questions Before You Read This Book

James A. Howenstine, MD

Do natural health solutions really exist?

Yes. Nutritious foods, vitamins, minerals, aminoacids, algae and extracts from herbs, plants, flowers, roots, seeds, bushes, trees, fish, mussels and animals have all been proven to have healing properties

If natural health solutions exist for many modern diseases, why don't the pharmaceutical companies produce them?

Pharmaceutical companies exist to make money. (As all companies do.) One company makes 90% of its profits from only 6 patented and skillfully marketed drugs. They cannot patent natural products, so there is no profit motive to provide these products.

Why don't more doctors know about natural health solutions?

The medical profession and pharmaceutical companies work together very closely.

We physicians continue our learning by reading medical journals and attending meetings. These are almost always oriented towards pharmaceutical companies and their drugs. The end result is the average physician has almost no awareness of the curative potential of natural treatments.

Why has there been, in some cases, a negative image regarding natural health solutions?

There's no question there has been some exaggeration and hype by untrained people talking about these issues. However, that doesn't take away from the effectiveness of natural health solutions, when carefully chosen by skilled professionals.

There seem to be so many natural health products out there, with all sorts of claims about them. It all seems pretty confusing to me.

I have carefully chosen and screened the premier natural health products we recommend and explain how to take them.

They work and I tell you *why* they work.

An Important Word About Side Effects

There are in general two kinds of therapies: pharmaceutical drugs and natural treatments.

Pharmaceutical drugs sometimes have unknown side effects which can be severe and only show up years later, after the damage is done. As one such example Baycol, a widely used cholesterol-lowering drug, was recently removed from the market after a number of deaths were linked to it.

This is a problem for some modern day pharmaceutical drugs. Their side effects can be unrecognized until used by large numbers of patients over a period of time.

In other cases, drugs will help solve one problem but create another. This is a dilemma I often faced as a doctor.

Natural treatments are much more in harmony with the body and work with it. In general, natural solutions have far fewer side effects than pharmaceutical drugs.

Where To Obtain The Natural Health Products I Recommend In This Book

Our own *Natural Health Team* offers many of the products mentioned in this book. However, whenever possible we offer you an *alternative* source where you can obtain them.

I recommend these products because they work. Your health is what is important, not whether you choose to obtain these natural health products from us or from someone else.

About Our *Natural Health Team*

We have created the Natural Health Team to be a reliable, independent source of information about natural health products *that work.*

I also welcome your questions. You may contact me with your questions or comments at: doctorjim@naturalhealthteam.com

We care about your health.

Dr. James A Howenstine
Natural Health Team

Internet: www.naturalhealthteam.com
Email: doctorjim@naturalhealthteam.com
Mailing Address: 7333 N.W. 54th St. Miami, Florida 33166

Table Of Contents

7

———————————

INTRODUCTION

My medical education was very conventional. I graduated from Northwestern University Medical School. We had a few lectures abut vitamins but very little information about nutrition. Because of lack of data about good nutrition and the woeful misinformation coming from supposed governmental authorities, many physicians still do not know what constitutes sound nutritional advice.

My mind set after finishing my residency training was that if there was no pharmaceutical drug to cure a disease, nothing helpful could be done. We doctors are often so pharmaceutically oriented that we are unaware that natural health solutions exist.

My choice to become a physician was a wonderful decision. There were no boring days! My patients taught me something new every day. There are fond memories of delightful hours teaching medical students, interns and residents. The challenges of caring for hospitalized patients were real, exciting, and often humbling. The strong friendships we often developed were a treasure to me.

Physicians in primary care (internal medicine, family practice, pediatrics, and obstetrics and gynecology) obtain 70% of the needed information from the interview with the patient and 30% from physical examination.

A male patient over 50 years of age should receive a rectal exam annually. This exam detects polyps and cancer in the rectal area, as well as disclosing enlargement of the prostrate gland and hard areas in the prostrate that may be sites of cancer. Women should have a breast and pelvic exam annually as well. Patients with heart and lung disease should have their hearts and lungs listened to on a regular basis. If your physician does not examine you regularly, consider changing physicians.

There has been an explosion in important medical knowledge in the 1990's. More and more, individuals are taking responsibility for their own health. These people buy products at local health food stores or on the Internet or mail order that they believe will help keep them healthy or restore health. In a recent year, the value of *natural* health care products sold in the U.S. was 30 billion dollars, surpassing the 27 billion dollars spent on pharmaceutical products. When a major change like this begins it is probably inexorable.

Physicians learn about advances in medical care from medical journals. Articles published in these journals typically contain very little information about natural health treatments. Additionally, medical journals are to a large extent subsidized by advertisements from pharmaceutical firms. It would take great personal courage to *publish an article about a natural therapy that could replace or cut earnings from a drug and thus potentially harm advertising revenue.*

When a natural health company has as effective product, they must be careful to downplay any claims about the product, as curative type claims are likely to be followed by closure and the need to spend a huge amount of money for long- term research to prove the product is truly beneficial.

In the August 2, 2001 issue of the New England Journal of Medicine there was a superb review article about Autoimmune Diseases, written by A. David and B. Diamond, MD. In the therapy section of this article there was not a single sentence about the ability of thymic extract combined with vitamins and minerals to arrest rheumatoid arthritis, systemic lupus erythematosis, psoriasis, multiple sclerosis, hepatitis B and hepatitis C. This lack of information about thymic extract was not malicious. There is a nearly total lack of awareness about natural treatments in the conventional medical community.

To prove the efficacy of a therapy usually requires enormous expense (up to two hundred million dollars) to fund long term, double blind studies. This type of funding is not available to an individual practitioner and even if available, *there is no guarantee that successful results would be published in a reputable journal because of the clear conflict of interest medical journals face in publishing articles that could hurt pharmaceutical sales and decrease advertising revenue.*

Pharmaceutical companies normally sell drugs that have been patented. *For this reason they have little interest in natural solutions that cannot be patented.* This certainly does not mean that these natural substances have no value. Just look at one example.

At one time in my practice, I had 5 patients with rheumatoid arthritis, which was so serious it could only be controlled with a drug called methotrexate. This drug is used primarily in chemotherapy and over long term usage there is a danger that the user will develop cancer because of injury to the bone marrow. Methotrexate was treating one problem and possibly creating another.

One day, I read about an extract from New Zealand mussels that was effective in rheumatoid arthritis. *After trying it for two months, all 5 of my patients were able to stop taking methotrexate.*

This experience changed my attitude toward natural health products forever and started me on my search for natural health solutions for our bodies. You will read about a variety of natural health products that work for specific diseases. Some of these treatments are simple and inexpensive. Humans have a psychological quirk that if it does not cost much, it cannot be any good. I urge you to avoid this manner of thinking which could cause you to miss several superb, inexpensive natural solutions.

Yes, pharmaceutical drugs have their place *and natural solutions have theirs.*

Try to open your mind as this book guides you to *natural* ways of dealing with health problems.

James A. Howenstine, MD

Chapter 1

Are There Problems With The Food We Eat And The Water We Drink?

It's a lot easier to stay healthy than to get healthy after becoming ill.

To stay healthy we have to start with the food we eat and the water we drink.

The soil our food comes from has been changed in our modern world. Chemical fertilizers have caused the protein content of vegetables to decrease and the vital trace minerals we need are no longer being replaced.

There is a striking difference in the quality of the food grown by the Amish in Lancaster County, for example, and the food produced by agribusiness. The Amish still use horse manure as fertilizer.

One consequence of the use of pesticides, chemical fertilizers and the disappearance of manure is that earthworms have been killed. This creates serious problems for the soil. Earthworms make canals in the soil that facilitates the dispersion of air and water throughout the soil. In the absence of earthworms, the soil tends to be less porous and water runs off instead of entering the soil. This produces erosion.

The second problem of lack of earthworms is the disappearance of the valuable nutrition to the soil provided by the excreta of the worms.

Dietary Supplementation With Vitamins, Minerals and Nutrients

One of the most critical things that an individual can do to improve his or her health is to ensure that you are obtaining a needed amount of vitamins, minerals, and nutrients on a daily basis. You can't get these from the normal food you eat, so you must get them from somewhere else. When we do not obtain these substances we are more vulnerable to narrowing of arteries (arteriosclerosis), diabetes, cancer, cataracts, and other serious health problems.

There are three general categories of vital substances that you must know about: vitamins, minerals, and nutrients. Many persons believe that *"vitamins are vitamins"* and that they are all basically the same. *Nothing could be further from the truth.*

Vitamins in tablet form often do not disintegrate in the intestinal tract, so the nutrients become lost in the stool. I have occasionally seen X-rays with un-dissolved vitamin tablets in the intestinal tract ready to pass from the body. One component often placed in vitamin preparations (DCP) is a binding agent needed to keep all the ingredients in one piece. DCP does not break up easily so the vitamin often passes out in the stool.

Conventional medical wisdom has always held that substances like DHP and added inert substances found in vitamins and pharmaceutical drugs are not absorbed through the gastrointestinal tract, so they pass out harmless in the stools. Researchers at the University of London found in experiments on rats that polystyrene particles were absorbed through the intestinal wall and appeared via the portal vein in the liver. This suggests that there may be few or no substances that will not enter the venous and lymphatic circulation to some degree, including aluminum and silicon.

Many pharmaceutical drugs contain "insoluble" additives. Another group of British scientists at St. Bartholomew's Hospital has discovered aluminum, silicon and titanium in pathologic specimens from patients with Crohn's Disease (regional ileitis). Dr. Emmanuel Libman suggested that Crohn's Disease might be caused by toothpaste, which, of course, contains silicon and aluminum as well as fluoride. Crohn's Disease is an inflammatory illness, which produces scarring in the small intestine that frequently leads to surgery for bowel obstruction.

Cut-rate vitamins often contain additives, food allergens, sugar, artificial food coloring, and flavoring. The potency and purity can vary from pill to pill within the same bottle. When tested, the pills may only manifest 60% of the claimed quantity of nutrient.

Expired products may be kept on the shelves hoping they will sell. Timed - release pills may fail to dissolve at the *appropriate location* in your body and the benefit is lost.

Synthetic vitamin E (dl-alpha tocopherol or dl-alpha-tocopheryl) is a byproduct of petroleum products (acetone and turpentine). *Natural vitamin E* (d-alpha-tocopherol or d-alpha-tocopheryl) is better absorbed, more active, persists longer, and gives better antioxidant support. The natural vitamin E is more expensive so many manufacturers use the less expensive, but less effective, synthetic products.

A vitamin program needs balance because some vitamins are able to cancel out the effects of others and too much of one substance may nullify the effect of another.

Vitamins in a significant dosage give valuable antioxidant protection which leads to a 20 to 40% reduction in cancer, heart disease, cataracts and other health problems. The needed vitamins include:

Vitamin A - 5,000 units, Beta-carotene - 15,000 units,

Vitamin C - several hundred to 2,000mg.,

Citrus Bioflavinoids - 100mgs.,

Vitamin D3 Cholecalciferol - 400 IU,

Vitamin E - 400IU,

Vitamin B1 (Thiamine) - 50mg.,

Folic Acid - 400 mcg.,

Biotin - 300mcg.,

Betaine HCL - 100mg., and

Pantothenic Acid - 100mg.

Mineral supplements are also important, particularly when we know the soil has been seriously depleted from lack of trace mineral replacement. Among the minerals needed are calcium, magnesium, phosphorus, potassium, iodine, zinc, copper, boron, manganese, chromium, selenium 200 mcg., vanadium and molybdenum.

The added nutrients should include Omega 3 fatty acids, either from flax oil or seed, perilla oil, or fish oil (eicosapentaenoic or docosahexaenic acid).

Additional valuable nutrients include PABA - 100mg., DL methionine - 100mg., Bromelain - 100mg., Choline - 90 mg., Chlorella, Rutin - 25 mg., and Silica (horsetail) - 15mg.

Loose powder, capsules or soft gels are the preferred way to administer vitamins, *not tablets.*

What About Vitamins?

Human bodies are incredibly complex and varied. To say that they need only 50 mg. of Vitamin C daily is ridiculous. This may be an amount sufficient to prevent scurvy, but it may be far less than that needed for maximum health. Dr. Linus Pauling thought that 10 grams a day was necessary.

A study at UCLA showed that people using 400 mg. or more of Vitamin C daily had only *half* the cardiac deaths and lived 8 years longer than those not taking Vitamin C.

Vitamin C is important in the synthesis of steroid hormones, absorption of iron, formation of bile, and the synthesis of nerve transmitters. It is vital in the production of collagen that forms the framework for bone, connective tissue, cartilage, and skin.

Vitamin C is an effective anti-oxidant in the water component parts of the body. It not only neutralizes free radicals but regenerates Vitamin E. Vitamin C is abundant in white blood cells that function to draw bacteria into the cell where they are destroyed by enzymes and free radicals. Vitamin C protects cells from injury in fighting off bacterial invaders. Other benefits of Vitamin C include production of interferon, which has antiviral properties and natural killer cells which are T lymphocytes that attack infected and cancerous cells. In addition Vitamin C blocks free radical damage to artery walls, increases HDL (good) cholesterol and lowers the level of lipoprotein(a), which adheres to damaged locations in artery walls.

Cancer begins when the DNA of a single cell is damaged and mutates into a cancer cell. This cell reproduces a colony of malignant cells. Our DNA takes tens of thousands of hits daily by free radicals, but cancer only appears when the immune system has been overwhelmed. Vitamin C helps protect cellular DNA from free radical damage and enhances the immune response to mop up these abnormal cells.

Population studies have shown that high consumption of Vitamin C from foods and supplements decreases the risk of cancer of the bladder, breast, cervix, colon, esophagus, mouth, lung, and pancreas.

Natural vitamins absorbed *from food* are superior to "supplemental" vitamins as they are attached to complexes that facilitate their absorption (Vitamin C with bioflavinoids).

The body does not manufacture vitamin C. The correct dosage need varies from person to person, but might lie between several hundred and 2000 mg. daily.

Vitamin D

Lack of Vitamin D has always been found among the elderly and the housebound. Deficiency of Vitamin D is related to higher rates of breast, ovary, colon, and prostate cancer; increased incidence of multiple sclerosis, progression of osteoarthritis, impairment of the immune response, high blood pressure and mood disorders.

Ultraviolet light initiates the conversion of a Vitamin D precursor in the skin to a substance that, after changes in the liver and kidneys, becomes the active form of Vitamin D. Sunscreens with a protection factor of 8 or more block 95% of Vitamin D production. With equal sun exposure, an 80 year old is able to create only 50% of the Vitamin D produced by an 8 year old.

In an important study from the March 19, 1998 New England Journal of Medicine, 290 patients admitted to Massachusetts General Hospital were studied for evidence of Vitamin D deficiency. 57% of these patients were found to be Vitamin D deficient and in 22% the deficiency was severe. In a subgroup of 77 healthy patients with an average age of 44 years, 42% were Vitamin D deficient and in 11% the lack was severe.

A surprising and disconcerting finding in this study was that 46% of those regularly taking vitamin supplements were found to be lacking adequate Vitamin D in their blood.

Some observers believe that the cause for this deficiency of Vitamin D *lies in inadequate exposure to sunlight.* I recommend that sunlight should be permitted into contact with the skin of the face and arms at least 15 to 30 minutes, three times weekly. Too much sun is harmful, of course, *but too little is equally bad.*

Vitamin D deficiency is not a problem in tropical countries where sun exposure is normal. The incidence of osteoporosis, hip and spinal fractures, cataracts, and colon and prostate cancer are also lower in the tropics.

A highly active form of Vitamin D has been isolated from butter and may explain why skin cancer is much less frequent in persons using butter when compared to those eating artificial margarine. Perhaps one reason for the rising frequency of skin cancer is the switch from natural butter to synthetic margarine.

Osteoporosis is now being diagnosed in women in their 40's. These patients exhibit intense bone pain, muscle weakness, and even difficulty in walking. *Women with fibromyalgia who have similar symptoms have been discovered to have lower than normal bone density, which is very suspicious of osteoporosis.* These patients need to be screened for Vitamin D deficiency with a blood Vitamin D level. Therapy is easy with Vitamin D and Calcium.

Another aspect of this problem is the estrogen dominance of all females and males living in developed nations. This always is accompanied by progesterone lack. The use of natural progesterone might be able to help these young women recover from osteoporosis and fibromyalgia. At this time, 20% of the patients in rheumatologists offices are suffering from fibromyalgia, which is a very common and very disabling problem for many women. Estrogen dominance will be discussed in more detail in Chapter 31 on Women's Health Issues.

Vitamin E

In a large population study, nurses taking 100 mg. of Vitamin E had a 50% reduction in heart deaths. The recommended dose of Vitamin E is only 10 mg. It is impossible to take in more than 25 mg of Vitamin E from food daily. Some authorities think that 800 mg. daily is the correct dose.

Folic Acid

Very few women of child bearing years are taking folic acid. This substance has been proven to prevent neural tube defects such as spina bifida and hydrocephalus, when taken in a dosage of 400 mcg. daily before pregnancy. If a person waits until pregnant the fetal abnormality is already established.

All women of child - bearing age who might become pregnant should be taking 400 mg. of folic acid.

Women taking 400 mcg. of folic acid also have a decreased risk of heart attack and protection against Alzheimer's Disease and stroke. After 15 years of 400 mcg. of folic acid there is a 75% reduction in the number of women who get colon cancer.

Recently it has become apparent that pharmaceutical drugs may *interfere* with the absorption or metabolism of many vitamins and minerals, causing important deficiencies. The inability to properly absorb Vitamin B 12 in persons taking the proton pump inhibitors Prevacid (lansoprazole) and Prilosec (omeprazole) is discussed in detail in Chapter 26 Dementia In The Elderly (Alzheimer's Disease).

If you are taking pharmaceutical medicines, the chart in **Appendix "A"**, will alert you to possible problems of your medicine interacting negatively with the essential vitamins and minerals. This is reprinted, courtesy of the Health Sciences Institute.

The Council for Responsible Nutrition surveyed 22,000 persons and there was not a single person who was able to get the 100% RDI (recommended daily intake) of vitamins from the food he or she was eating. *This means that everyone needs supplemental vitamins.*

Starting a vitamin, mineral, and nutrient program starts a person on the road to better health. Your body has a greater capability to cope with environmental pollutants and your immune system can start to protect you from arterial damage, cancer, diabetes and arthritis in a greatly enhanced manner. We recommend Mega Multi supplement. Obtain this from Natural Health Team. Phone 1-800-4162806.

Fiber

Dr. Dennis Burkett of South Africa studied the eating habits of tribal natives and those of the Caucasians living in South Africa. He had observed that the natives did not have diverticulitis, which was a common problem in the whites. He also noted that the natives had a diet of fruit and vegetables, in contrast to the "modern" food of the whites.

The reason for the difference was that the native diet was very high in fiber. Everything eaten by the natives was eliminated within 24 hours whereas food in the modern, western diet often remained in the individual several days before elimination.

He popularized the taking of 2 or more tablespoons of oat bran daily to improve elimination in persons eating the western diet. Flax seed appears to have considerably more fiber than oat bran and should accomplish the same benefits.

Fermented Foods

Our ancestors ate fermented foods containing lactobacilli on a regular basis. Foods such as sauerkraut and yogurt containing bacilli keep the population of dangerous bacteria in the colon at low levels so they cannot cause a disease.

However, when an antibiotic is taken, the antibiotic *kills* the good lactobacilli and allows the disease producing e. coli 0157:117, salmonella, and Candida (yeast) to proliferate and be able to cause a serious illness. Taking a few tablespoons of sauerkraut or yogurt daily (be sure it has not been pasteurized, which kills the bacteria) can be *very* beneficial to our health.

These "good " bacteria from fermenting cabbage and milk create agents that have powerful effects in preventing and even possibly treating cancer.

The Problem Of Margarine and Hydrogenated Fats

Margarine is an *artificial* product, as are the hydrogenated fats (safflower, corn, sunflower, canola, and soy), which are used in cooking and for salad oil. In the process of manufacturing these, oils are heated to high temperatures and treated with chemicals. The end product of hydrogenation is margarine, *which is chemically very close to plastic.* Would you eat plastic? Of course not. But each time you eat margarine you are closer to eating plastic than you think. Salad oils have the same problem.

These Fats Create Serious Problems For Our Bodies.

They have *no* nutritional value.

In the process of clearing this *plastic sludge* from our body, many free radicals are created which stress our body to get rid of.

Margarine is probably partially responsible for the increasing problem of heart attacks in nations that have switched from lard or butter to margarine for cooking.

The breakdown of the abnormal fats raise LDL (bad cholesterol) and this gets deposited into artery walls leading to greatly increased levels of heart disease.

The switch to margarine has been associated with rapidly rising levels of melanoma and skin cancer. Butter contains a component that prevents the development of skin cancer.

These hydrogenated fats could be considered *slow poison*. You do not drop dead like you would with cyanide but your arteries and ability to fight cancer gets impaired, so you die at 62 instead of in an auto accident at age 82.

The Present Essential Fatty Acid Crisis

The body cannot make vital omega 3 and omega 6 fatty acids. Omega 3 fatty acid can be found in flax oil, perilla oil and fish. Omega 6 fatty acid is found in safflower, sunflower, canola, soybean, corn, hemp, pumpkin, and sesame seeds, nuts and oils.

The proper ratio between Omega 6 and Omega 3 fatty acids should be about 4:1. Currently this ratio is heavily skewed toward omega 6 at 20:1 to 25:1. This harmful imbalance has been brought about by the massive use of synthetic vegetable oils in our foods. Unfortunately, all these oils are synthetic transfats, which makes them health risks. Omega 3 fatty acids are unsuitable for salad dressing as they quickly become rancid.

Our meat is from cattle grown on corn instead of grazing. Grazed animals have 5 times more omega 3 fatty acids than corn fed cattle. A second problem is that catfish, salmon, trout, and shrimp are being farmed. These fish eat omega 6 grains instead of minnows, drill, algae, and insects, which are rich in omega 3 fatty acids. This results in seafood that has much less omega 3 than native seafood. .

Mother's milk has abundant Omega 3 fatty acid in the form of Docosahexaenoid acid (DHA). *The absence of DHA in commercial formula milk may be contributing to the rising incidence of attention deficit disorder and hyperactivity (ADHD) seen in children.*

Consequences of inadequate balances of Omega 3 and 6 fatty acids

- Omega 6 fatty acids promote inflammation and omega 3 fatty acids retard inflammation.

- Food, airborne allergies, and asthma will increase.

- Heart disease will increase.

- Weakened immune systems will increase.

This problem can be corrected by ingestion of flax, perilla and fish oil.

Flaxseed

Many authorities consider flaxseed as *nature's perfect food.* Germany consumes 60,000 tons of flaxseed annually in bread, cakes, and cereals.

Lignans

Flaxseed has a very high amount of lignans, between 100 and 800 times more than that available from wheat bran, soybeans, and oatmeal. Lignans are phytochemicals found in the cell matrix of plants. These flax lignans are important because of antiviral, anti-fungal, and antibacterial properties. *Flax lignans also have a vital role in helping prevent cancer.*

Estrogen is a suspected risk factor for breast cancer. Lignans are converted in the intestine to a form that binds to estrogen receptors. They also increase the production in the body of sex binding globulins, which remove excess estrogen from the body.

A Finnish study in the 1980's found that women with breast cancer had low levels of lignans in their urine and women who did not have breast cancer had much higher levels of lignans in their urine.

Fiber

Flaxseed (linseed) is an excellent source of dietary fiber. *Fiber corrects constipation, softens the stool and helps remove cholesterol.*

Amino Acids

Flaxseed contains all the essential amino acids, which the body must obtain from the diet.

Minerals

Flaxseed contains all the major minerals and many of the trace minerals.

Linseed Oil

The oil pressed from flaxseed contains 50 to 60% linolenic acid and 15 to 25% linoleic acid. Both these must be obtained from the diet, but only linolenic acid is very deficient in the modern U.S. diet.

Flax oil improves metabolism and is often associated with weight loss.

Flax oil is converted into prostaglandins, which regulate heart function, blood pressure, and function of arteries.

Flax oil has an important role to play in treating cancer, arthritis, diabetes, arteriosclerosis, high blood pressure, and immune disorders.

Omega 3 and omega 6 fatty acids form the membranes surrounding every cell.

Flaxseed needs to be eaten without heating as heat destroys the beneficial enzymes and converts the oil to a bad transfat.

Grinding small quantities of flaxseed and storing a two or three day residual in the refrigerator ensures the nutritional benefits of flax oil are intact.

Flaxseed varies between 33% and 43% oil. Between 15% and 25% of this oil is linoleic acid and 50 to 60% of the oil is linolenic acid. This is wonderful because linolenic acid is not as readily available from food as the other essential fatty acid linoleic acid is. Flax oil also contains beta carotene (precursor to Vitamin A), Vitamin E, lecithin and phosphatides, all of which are needed for efficient digestion of fats and oils.

Flaxseed, flax oil, and ground flaxseed can be obtained from your local health food store and from Natural Health Team. Phone 1-800-4162806

Magnesium

Magnesium deficiency is very common, particularly in elderly persons. Approximately 60% of this mineral is found in our bones and 26% in muscles, with the remainder in soft tissue and body fluids. The tissues with the highest concentrations of magnesium are those that are very active in metabolism (brain, heart, kidneys, and liver).

Magnesium is essential for many principal biologic processes, including metabolism of glucose, production of cellular energy, and synthesis of nucleic acids and protein. It is also vital for the electrical stability of cells, maintenance of membrane integrity, muscular contraction, nerve conduction, and the regulation of vascular tone. Magnesium supplementation may be of greater importance than calcium.

Magnesium is involved with regulation of acid base balance, helps promote absorption of minerals including calcium, phosphorus, sodium, and potassium. Magnesium helps utilization of B complex vitamins, Vitamin C, and Vitamin E. It aids in bone growth and is necessary for proper function of muscles.

Many foods contain magnesium, which is found primarily in green vegetables but is also present in wheat germ, soybeans, milk, whole grains, seafood, figs, corn, apples and oil rich seeds and nuts. All this makes it hard to understand why most people are deficient of magnesium. However, only 30 to 40% of ingested food magnesium is absorbed *and high calcium intake, alcohol, surgery, diuretics, liver disease, kidney disease and oral contraceptives all decrease magnesium absorption.*

In the past, water was a good source of magnesium but concerns about lead, cadmium, fluoride and other toxins in water have led many people to either drink filtered water or bottled water, which has very little magnesium.

The U.S. Department of Agriculture states that only 25% of Americans have a magnesium intake that meets USRDA standards. A global pattern of large numbers of sudden cardiac deaths has emerged, which have arrthymias and many are believed to be caused by magnesium deficiency. In the U.S. alone 8 million deaths between 1940 and 1994 are thought to be due to magnesium deficiency.

In a Swedish study, 27 municipalities had their drinking water investigated between 1969 and 1978. The mortality from arteriosclerotic (ischemic) heart disease was inversely related to the magnesium content of their water. This was particularly valid for men. These researchers concluded that high magnesium content in water reduces the risk for death from ischemic heart disease. This study has been confirmed in U.K., Netherlands, Finland, Russia, India and other nations.

In one study in the U.S., in 1959 100 persons with heart disease (one third had heart attacks) were given imtramuscular injections of Magnesium Sulfate .5 to 1.0 grams every 5 days for 12 injections. There was only one death. In the preceding year when no magnesium was used, there was a 30% death rate in 196 similar heart patients. Similar results have been confirmed from South Africa.

The population studies showing better survival rates in areas where the water has high magnesium levels suggest that high magnesium intake from water is saving lives in persons who have narrowed arteries to the heart. The difference in death rates probably relates to higher levels of magnesium in the blood, protecting hearts from ventricular fibrillation (sudden death) when episodes of cardiac ischemia (heart attack) occur.

One problem in medicine is that physicians will read about or hear about a new idea and all agree that it has merit. However, physicians are busy and get distracted Many believe that magnesium protects the heart from sudden death, but this concept has never been instituted.

In a hospital emergency room setting, a person entering with severe chest pain may have a cardiac problem, esophageal spasm, or gall bladder attack, along with several other possible conditions. Those who do turn out to have a heart attack will probably have a higher survival rate if given an injection of magnesium immediately, in the emergency room.

Bone tissue is alive, complex, dynamic and has a wide range of nutritional needs. Magnesium may play as critical a role in bone formation and maintenance as does calcium. High calcium intake, without additional magnesium, actually *inhibits magnesium absorption.*

Osteoporotic bones in women who were depleted of magnesium had fragile calcium crystals in their bones, whereas osteoporotic women with normal magnesium levels had normal calcium crystals in their bones.

Magnesium supplements have prevented the formation of calcium oxalate crystals, the most common cause of kidney stones.

Magnesium has been helpful in the therapy of premenstrual syndrome. Many women with this problem have high sugar and high dairy fat intakes, both of which lower magnesium values in the blood. Supplemental magnesium appears to be a necessity, particularly in persons who are getting little magnesium from their water.

How Safe Is Fructose?

High fructose corn syrup came into widespread use as a sugar substitute in the 1970's because of its lower price. By 1990 the quantity of fructose consumed had gone up ten fold. This is now present in candy, soda, cereal, crackers, bread and hundreds of other foods.

Fructose was believed to be a safe sugar substitute because it has no adverse effects on either blood sugar values or insulin output. However, there are two serious problems from fructose usage.

When ingested, fructose is immediately shuttled directly to the liver. In the liver it is a key building block in the manufacture of triglycerides. These triglycerides are then transported to the bloodstream carried by LDL (bad) cholesterol to the arteries where they deposit in the artery walls. Animal research has shown that feeding a high fructose diet to animals is one of the fastest ways to raise triglyceride levels in the blood. *The amount of fructose eaten by Americans is comparable in quantity to that fed to these animals.*

Fructose is commonly regarded as the sugar found in fruit. The important distinction is that in fruit the quantity of fructose is small and it is bound to complex plant fiber, nutrients and minerals. In this way, fructose containing fruit and vegetables are a valuable protection against cardiovascular disease and other health problems.

The second major problem with fructose is its ability to combine with amino acids to form advanced glycation end products (AGEs). AGEs are believed to be permanent. They accumulate in body tissues where they accelerate aging and thus contribute to the formation of cataracts, narrowing of arteries and kidney disease.

High intake of fructose contributes to increased levels of glycation in the body. Reducing all sugar intake appears to be a wise health measure.

Brown Rice

The removal of the outer portion of the grain of rice to create a more appealing white rice has had serious nutritional consequences. Rice is a basic staple food for much of the world. Thiamine and other key ingredients have been removed from the white rice grain. Certainly, the world's health would be greatly benefited if it were no longer removed. Powerful nutrients have recently been discovered in the husk of rice. Everyone should be eating brown rice.

High Protein Diet

The average person in the U.S. eats too much protein. The dietary estimates are that we eat 100 to 150 grams of protein daily. This has several undesirable consequences:

High protein intake plays a major role in the causation of osteoporosis. Countries that eat far less protein and obtain calcium from vegetable sources have far less osteoporosis.

A high protein intake is usually high in fat and high fat intakes are a recognized contributing factor for the development of various cancers.

The high protein intake places a strain on the kidneys to eliminate the byproducts of protein metabolism and increases the frequency of gout.

Good health can be maintained with a protein intake of 50 grams for women and 60 grams daily for men.

Homogenized Milk

In the process of homogenizing milk the fat molecules are broken up making them easy to absorb. The enzyme xanthine oxidase travels along with the fat particles and has a deleterious action on arteries.

Skim milk has no fat so it is not homogenized. Therefore, drinking skim milk and adding pure cream to the milk container whenever you need a richer milk seems to be a safer way to use milk.

What Should Be Done About Our Food?

Eat lots of fresh vegetables and fruit, organically grown if possible. An example of how tasty vegetables can be is a recipe called Taj Mahal Spread.

This is a wonderful hors d'oeuvres for entertaining and my wife and I like it with soup at lunch.

1 cup of dried lentils

1 cup dried split peas

1/3 cup plus three tablespoons olive oil

1 cup chopped red onion (white works fine but the red onion gives a sweeter taste)

2 tablespoons chopped garlic (puree it)

2 teaspoons of ground cumin (I put three and prefer whole cumin)

1 cup (packed) fresh cilantro

2 tablespoons of fresh lemon juice

1 teaspoon chili powder

salt and pepper to taste

Cook lentils and split peas in large pot of boiling salt water until very tender about 35 minutes (better cooked apart since lentils cook much faster). Drain.

Heat 1/3 cup of oil in heavy large skillet over medium heat. Add onion and garlic and sauté until onion is translucent about 5 minutes. Add cumin and stir 1 minute. Transfer mixture to processor. Add lentils, split peas, cilantro, lemon juice, chili powder, and remaining 3 tablespoons of oil. Process until smooth. Season generously with salt and pepper.

(Can be prepared a day ahead. Cover and refrigerate. Bring to room temperature before serving.)

Serve with pita bread.

Recipe thanks to Jean Michel and Suzanne Herrera.

Eat several servings of fish weekly. Reduce meat intake and keep cuts lean. Bake and broil instead of frying. Remove skin from chicken. When broiling hamburger and other meat turn every minute. This prevents searing of the meat and ensures uniform heating. Seared meat has carcinogenic protein.

A good general rule to follow about food would be to eat only food that spoils. Eat it before it spoils, of course. Following this rule will eliminate all dangerous processed food. *Ninety per cent of the money spent on food in the United States goes to buy processed food.*

Try to get several tablespoons of fermented food (yogurt or sauerkraut) into your diet daily.

Strongly consider eating Spirulina (Hawaii), Royal jelly, and Bee pollen.

These are packed with nutrients (amino acids, carotinoids, etc) and can be considered nearly perfect foods.

Eat raw food in the form of juicing or direct consumption of raw carrots, tomatoes, garlic, radishes, onions and olives. Many authorities believe that the ideal diet should contain 70 to 80% raw food. This includes food that has not been heated above 120 degrees F. Enzymes are destroyed by cooking and this contributes to problems with digestion of food.

A wonderful tasting juice recipe that provides valuable enzymes can be made from beets, carrots, apples, and ginger. Take 10 to 12 medium sized carrots (organic, if possible), one medium beet, one or two apples, and a 3/4 inch slice of fresh ginger root. Wash and cut before juicing. This will make one quart of juice.

Eat lots of garlic and onions.

Eat nuts that are not covered with synthetic vegetable oils.

Get plenty of fiber from fruit, vegetables, whole grain bread and cereals, and salads.

Use sea salt for seasoning and cooking instead of commercial salt and you will receive magnesium, calcium, potassium, sulfur, and trace minerals as well as sodium.

Avoid all sweeteners except stevia.

How Safe Is Aspartame (NutraSweet)?

Dr. Russell Blaycock, a neursurgeon at the Medical Univerisity of Mississippi, has written a book titled *Exitotoixins: The Taste That Kills,* which thoroughly explores the information about aspartame. Exitotoxins are substances that case hyperexcitation of brain cells so they fire their impulses very rapidly. They continue to do this until the brain cell becomes exhausted and may die. Normally, the exciting substances such as glutamate and aspartate are transmitting substances which permit communicationbetween brain cells. These compounds are so toxic that *the body keeps them at very low brain levels.* Any substance that increases the levels of these substances has the potential to kill brain cells andc cause degeneration of brain and spinal cord.

Human beings are primarily exposed to exitotoxins as food additives. The most widely known is monosodium glutamate (MSG) which can be found in hydrolyzed vegetable protein, vegetable proten, soy isolate and Chinese food.

Aspartame or Nutrasweet is composed of two amino acids, phenylalanine and aspartic acid. The aspartic acid is as powerful as an exitotoxin as is glutamate. Phenylalanine is known to produce seizures and act as a neurotoxin in the brain. Normally, the amino acids are part of proteins which are slowly broken down by the body so the level in the brain always remains at low levels. When a sweetener contains high amounts of these isolated amino acids the brain level may, after ingestion, become high enough to cause brain cell death, seizures and death.

Aspartame contains aspartic acid which is just as toxic as glutamate. Three powerful neurotoxins are found in aspartame. One of these, methanol, is widely known to cause blindness by injuring the optic nerves. The level of methanol permitted in aspartame is 7 times higher than the quantity permitted in other foods. The second toxin, aspartic acid, is an exitotoxin which produces cullular excitation capable of leading to cell death. *In new born babies whose mothers use aspartame permanent changes in brain formation occur that lead to behavioral problems and hyperactivity. The third toxin phenylalanine lowers the seizure threshold making convulsions more likely.*

High levels of phenylalanine and aspartic acid have been documented in brain tissue. Phenylalanine accumulates in very high amounts in the hypothalamus, which regulates the endocrine system, autonomic nervous system, sleep /wake cycles, appetite and the emotional system.

In patients with multiple sclerosis when the disease flares up the protective membrane around the nerve fibers (myelin) breaks down permitting blood substances to enter the brain. In this manner blood containing high levels of aspartic acid, phenylalanine and methanol could seep through these holes and enter the brain. Any person with asymptomatic multiple sclerosis can break out with full blown MS after exposure to aspartame. Furthermore, persons consuming large quantities of NutraSweet can develop symptoms of MS because of the toxic agents in NutraSweet.

Three American Airline pilots who were heavy users of aspartame have died. One had a stroke. Others have developed disorientation, blindess and dizziness (vertigo) and were found to have low blood sugar values (hypoglycemia). The toxic effects of exitotoxins are greatly mangnifed by the presence of hypoglycemia. A pilot who skips breakfast will become slightly hungry and weak from low blood sugar. However, if he has also taken NutraSweet his hypoglycemia and exitotoxins exposure may produce confusion, blurred vision, disorientation and vertigo. Brain cells need gluose to function and coma may appear in hypoglycemic situations.

Human subjects are often at excess risk both from aspartame, which is frequently consumed several times daily, along with MSG and hydrolyzed vegetable protein.

Aspartame has been proven to cause seizures in research studies on human subjects. The simultaneous ingestion of Crystal Light and NutraSweet has often caused seizures. One man who had an abnormal vein deep in his brain stopped having seizures when he stopped using aspartame and Crystal Light. The lowering of the seizure threshold seen with aspartame may permit seizures to appear in persons with small brain scars from a difficult childbirth or brain injury who would have lived their lives seizure free without the aspartame usage.

A four year old child was drinking aspartame sweetened root beer when he went beserk. The child became hyperactive, violent and complained of headache. No new headaches appeared off NutraSweet but the mother was skeptical so she allowed the child to use aspartame again. The same symptoms reappeared.

Dr. Freider and Grimm did a study in Israel where they fed pregnant mice an excitotoxin. The offspring had normal learning for simple things *but exhibited severe impairment when tested for complex tasks*. Study of their brains disclosed *the neurotrasmitter acetyl choline was 80 % reduced and continued to be reduced during the whole childhood of the animal.*

These findings in mice suggest that profound changes occur in the brain chemistry of children that are exposed to exitotoxins during fetal development. Dr. Louis Elsas testified before Congress that *aspartame is a neurotoxin that triggers birth defects*. Can these changes be reversed? Massive doses probably produce permanent cell death, particularly in the hypothalamus. Lesser dosage permits permanent recovery when aspartame is stopped. Continued long term usage may cause pernanent behavioral changes. Pregnant women often use diet soda during pregnancy to attempt to prevent weight gain. Pregnant mothers should not use aspartame and children should stop taking this toxic agent.

Take a multivitamin. Be sure the multivitamin does not contain iron. Iron in the pills can mask a serious iron deficiency and cause a delay in the diagnosis of iron deficiency anemia. Iron deficiency anemia frequently is caused by serious conditions such as cancer and ulcers that are slowly bleeding and should be discovered as quickly as possible. Don't cover it up with iron in your vitamins.

Of great importance also is that the taking of iron can make an individual with the metabolic problem of hemachromatosis much worse.

Hemachromatosis is a common metabolic abnormality, more frequent in males, that is unfortunately under diagnosed. Persons with this disease absorb too much iron from their diet and the deposition of this iron causes scarring in the liver, heart, pancreas, skin and testes.

These persons will obviously get into trouble sooner if they are taking iron in a supplement.

The most serious problem with having iron in a vitamin supplement is that supplemental iron appears to triple the risk of sustaining a heart attack.

What Can We Safely Use To Cook Food?

This is a very important question for the prevention of disease and maintenance of your health. One ready answer would be butter. This is a natural product. Margarine is an artificial product, has little nutritional value and is very difficult for the body to process and discharge.

The second cooking agent I recommend is virgin olive oil, which works well and is completely safe if you avoid high temperatures. Adding water as you cook keeps the temperature lower and avoids creating dangerous transfats.

The third choice would be lard. This was used for many years by our grandparents and is safe if it does not contain pesticides, which collect in fat tissue. Research to find out whether lard has pesticide residue could be very helpful.

A fourth cooking agent that is completely safe is coconut oil. This was commonly used in the past, but now appears to be available only in small quantities in health food stores.

Olive oil has two important components that completely stop the oxidation of LDL (bad cholesterol). These two compounds are destroyed in over-processed olive oil. Therefore, buy only virgin cold-pressed olive oil for cooking. This is more expensive, but more effective.

Whenever possible bake and broil instead of frying. When broiling meat such as hamburgers turn them every minute. This will prevent the meat from getting seared. The seared, blackened meat contains protein that has been badly damaged by excessive heat. This seared meat protein is the portion that has the carcinogens that we need to keep out of our bodies.

It is time for everyone to consider discontinuing the use of margarines, shortening and vegetable oils that are not real food and have great long-term adverse consequences for our health.

Unexpected Culinary Dangers

Microwaves give off high-energy electromagnetic waves that bombard food. This unnatural process creates abnormal amino acids and fatty acids that may be very toxic. An unpublished report disclosed that animals fed microwave food rapidly perished.

Plasticizers are substances added to plastics to produce a soft product, which feels better to the touch. These softeners are usually phthalates, which have the capability of separating from the plastic and entering our food and beverages. Pthalates are toxic to the liver, kidneys and reproductive organs.

Mediterranean Diet

This is an ideal diet for cardiac patients and would probably be good for everyone. This diet could be divided into 3 component parts.

Foods Eaten A Few Times Each Month

Red meat from cattle that are grazed and not exposed to hormones, antibiotics or pesticides from feed.

Foods Eaten A Few Times Each Week

Eggs, Poultry, Fish and Sweets. Avoid all use of white (refined) sugar, white flour and white rice, which are artificial products.

After refining, sugar has pharmacologic properties and is no longer a food.

The refining process greatly accelerates the movement of sugar into the blood stream by removing the fiber from the sugar cane. The body responds to this rapid rise in blood sugar by rapidly releasing large amounts of insulin into the blood to correct the sudden high sugar levels. This causes artery damage, high cholesterol and weight gain, secondary to depositing fat.

In an interesting experiment the sugar from one soft drink was able to damage the white blood cells' ability to ingest and kill gonococcal bacteria for 7 hours. This impaired immune function gives another reason to avoid eating or drinking refined (white) sugar.

Soft drinks also contain large quantities of phosphorus which when excreted pulls calcium out of the bones. Heavy users of soft drinks will have osteoporosis along with their damaged arteries.

Foods Eaten Daily

Fruits, beans, nuts, legumes, vegetables, brown rice, couscous, polenta, bulghur, whole grain bread, other grains, potatoes and natural cheese (straight from the farmer with no additives). Wheat processed becomes white flour, a nearly worthless substance from the health standpoint. In the same way, a good almond can become dangerous when treated with hydrogenated oil.

The benefits of this diet will be discussed in more detail in Chapter 4 on Heart Diseases.

Flax oil and perilla oil: Consider improving your Omega 3 fatty acid levels with daily ingestion of either flax or perilla oil. Much more about these substances will be discussed in Chapter 12 on Malignancies.

What Are The Problems Of Water?

Contamination with bacteria and parasites.

Waterborne illnesses kill 13 million people around the world each year. Milwaukee and Crater Lake, Oregon have had serious epidemics due to infectious agents in the water.

Contamination with petrochemical residue

Contamination with metals (lead, mercury, aluminum, fluoride)

The city of San Jose, California had a mini-epidemic of congenital abnormalities in children that was connected to Silicon Valley firms discharging used metals into the water, which contaminated the water table of San Jose.

Fluoridation

Fluoride occurs naturally as calcium fluoride. The bonding of fluoride with calcium is strong. The fluoride added to drinking water, however, is sodium fluoride, sodium silicofluoride, or hydrofluosilic acid. These three fluoride forms, when added to water, are far more toxic then calcium fluoride because their bonding to fluoride is easily broken, permitting the fluoride to seek bone and cause damage. Animal experiments have shown that the lethal dose of drinking water fluoride is 50 times less than that of calcium fluoride.

The U.S. Environmental Protection Agency has classified fluoride as more toxic than lead but less toxic than arsenic.

Does Fluoridation Decrease Tooth Decay?

Surprisingly, the evidence for decreasing cavities after fluoridation is not strong.

Most of Europe does not fluoridate water. The number of decayed, missing or filled teeth (DMF) in U.S. children twelve years old declined by 25% between 1974 and 1988. In the Netherlands, Sweden, and Finland, nations not using fluoride, the decline in DMF for the same years in twelve year olds was 36%, 40%, and 47% respectively.

In a study of 26,000 school children in Tucson, Arizona, Dr.Cornelius Steelink Emeritus Professor from the Department of Chemistry at the University of Arizona, discovered that the more fluoride a child drank, the more cavities occurred. His study suggested that decay was also related to low family income, bad diet, poor oral hygiene, and lack of access to dental care.

Some children drinking fluoridated water develop an unsightly staining of their teeth called dental fluorosis, which leads to psychological problems in some of these children.

One of the unfortunate problems with fluoride is that it accumulates in the body, with the body having no good mechanism for removal.

Could The Daily Drinking Of Fluoride Be Contributing To The Rising Incidence Of Cancer In The United States?

A population study in the U.S.A. compared the 10 largest cities fluoridating their water with the 10 largest cities that did not fluoridate their water. Both city groups had identical cancer rates before the study.

After a 20-year follow up, the cities fluoridating their water had 10%

more cancer than the cities not using fluoride. When this information was released, Dr. Dean Burk, the Chief Chemist Emeritus of U.S. National Cancer Institute, stated: *"In point of fact, fluoride causes more human death, and causes it faster, than any other chemical."*

Dr. Perry Cohn of the New Jersey Department of health did a survey of osteosarcoma (OS), a childhood cancer and the exposure to fluoride. This study showed that the rate of osteosarcoma in fluoride drinking boys below the age of 10 was 4.6 times greater than non fluoride drinking males of the same age. In the 10 to 19 age group, the rate of OS was 3.5 times higher for those drinking fluoride. In the over 20 to age 49 group, the ratio was more than two times higher in those drinking fluoride (Irish Medical Journal vol. 93 Number 6 September 2000).

Using the same level of fluoride as that placed in U.S. water, researchers at Nippon Dental School were able to show the transformation of normal cells into cancer cells.

Strong consideration should be given to the removal of fluoride from the water in those communities that are placing fluoride in their water.

Estrogen- like chemical pesticides reaches the groundwater and play a role in the rising incidence of breast cancer.

Chlorinated water has been incriminated as the primary cause of bladder cancer and possibly colon cancer.

High levels of lead, leaching off water pipes in some schools and homes, seems linked to permanent behavioral problems and decreased IQ in children.

Rainwater is contaminated with crop pesticides. Dr. Stephen Muller, a chemist at the Swiss General Institute for Environmental Science and Technology reports that much rainwater is contaminated with pesticides. Common pesticides such as atrazine, alachlor and others evaporate after being sprayed on a field. They then combine with water vapor in clouds.

When this vapor falls to earth as rain it falls everywhere, not just in fields.

Tests have shown that 9 of 41 storms had excessive levels of atrazine per liter. 100 nanograms per liter is the level regarded as borderline. One sample had 4000 ng. per liter, 40 times in excess of the safe limit.

Non Hodgkin's Lymphoma (NHL)

Research from Sweden has disclosed that both Americans and Europeans who contract Non Hodgkin's Lymphoma were 2.3 times more likely to have been exposed to the herbicide glyphose than individuals who did not have NHL. Glyphosates are non- selective systemic chemicals found in the popular weed killers ROUNDUP, EAZY WEEDER, AND SLAM. They kill weeds and grains, so are only suitable in yards.

What Appears To Be The Best Solution For The Many Problems Of Water?

My initial reaction was to suggest the use of distilled water. However, further investigation has disclosed that while better, this is not completely safe. Distilled water absorbs carbon dioxide from the air, making the water acidic. To neutralize this chronic intake of an acidic substance, the body needs to buffer the acid with calcium, potassium, magnesium and other alkaline minerals. This would lead to depletion of these key minerals over a period of time.

Long time users of distilled water have been reported to exhibit loss of clumps of hair (alopecia). This hair loss is a well recognized complication of iron lack or under active function of the thyroid gland.

I am not qualified to recommend which filtration system is best for you. In our home, we use the British Berkefeld water filter. Missionaries and relief workers being sent into remote or diseased areas of the world have used this for more than 100 years. The current model uses a ceramic filter that is wonderful in screening out bacterial and parasitic contaminants in the water. Chlorine and solvents are also removed.

The core of the filter is diatomaceous earth. The current filter has an activated carbon filter, which removes chemical and organic compounds.

Water filtered through a solid charcoal filter emerges slightly alkaline, which is ideal for good health. Water filtered by reverse osmosis is neutral and would be safe, if mineral supplements are taken to replace those removed.

Chapter 2

What Are The Additives In Our Food Doing To Our Health?

The average American now eats 9 pounds of chemicals annually. The list of foreign materials in our food includes additives, preservatives, dyes, bleaches, emulsifiers, antioxidants, flavors, buffers, noxious sprays, acidifiers, alkalizers, deodorants, moisturizers, anti-caking and anti-foaming agents, conditioners, curers, hydrolizers, hydrogenators, drying agents, gases, extenders, thickeners, sweeteners, maturers, fortifiers, *margarine, shortening, salad and cooking oils* .

In the advanced nations, the increased incidence of degenerative diseases (cancer, cardiovascular disease, diabetes, multiple sclerosis, and diseases of the liver and kidney) *has paralleled the increased consumption of unnatural, chemically altered fats.*

57% of our dietary fat consumption comes from commercially manufactured fats and oils, including margarine, shortening, salad and cooking oils. These are synthetic, dangerous substances.

In 1900, cancer killed one person out of 30. *It now kills one person in five.* In 1900, heart disease killed one person in every seven. Deaths from heart disease now include one out of every two persons.

Korean War autopsy studies revealed that young healthy soldiers dying in combat had an 80% incidence of early damage to their coronary arteries and 20% had more serious narrowing. *Clearly, something is very wrong with the U.S. lifestyle.*

Of the 60.000 chemicals in general use, *fewer than 2% have been tested for safety.* There are 5,000 known chemical additives. Of this group, one third are known to be safe. One third are generally regarded as safe. The *remaining one third have never been tested.*

One problem this widespread exposure to chemicals is creating is allergic reactions to the chemicals.

Colorants

Between the years 1940 and 1977, the quantity of colorants and additives in U.S. food increased *ten fold.*

In 1957, ten of thirteen dyes certified for use in food were found to cause cancer when injected below the skin of rats. It was estimated that a human would absorb twice the proportional quantity of dye when eaten, that the rat absorbed when injected subcutaneously. *The oil soluble colors were so toxic to rats that they died before studies could be completed to learn if the dyes were carcinogenic.*

Yellow AB and Yellow OB, which are known carcinogens, have been used to color margarine and butter. They are made from beta-napthylamine, which is known to be not toxic *but is also very carcinogenic.*

The commonly used food colors amaranth (red), bordeaux (brown) and procean (scarlet) are derived by compounding nitrogen with benzene (a distillate of coal).

Spices are often treated with fumigants or extracted with solvents.

Pesticides

DDT came into use to prevent infestation of crops with insects. Over time, it became clear that DDT, when stored in body fat, took many years to be eliminated. Nobel Prize Laureate Dr. Otto Warburg warned that a poison like DDT that interfered with cellular respiration causes irreparable harm and produces degenerative diseases such as cancer.

DDT was found in food fed to convicts in a federal prison. DDT remained in a plot of ground so easily that after seven years study, 80% of the DDT applied was still present. One of the replacements for DDT chlordane is *four times more toxic.*

A recent study of the insecticide diazinon disclosed that in families with a dog, following lawn treatment *the levels of air and carpet diazinon inside the home were 50 times higher than levels outside the home.* The levels of pesticide on the dog paws were between 55 and 250 times higher than levels found in the yard. Insecticide chemicals contain carbamates, or organophosphates. These chemicals kill insects by disrupting their nervous systems. The ability to form cholinesterase is inhibited and nerve impulses cannot be transmitted. Mammals, including humans, have the *same* neurotransmitters and experience the same breakdown in their nervous system after exposure to carbamates and organophosphates.

Is there any evidence of this damage in humans? Unfortunately the answer is yes.

Parkinson's Disease afflicts 1 million people in the U.S.A. Two percent of persons over 65 have this disease.

A population study from Denmark revealed that individuals working in the agriculture and horticulture industries had a high risk for developing Parkinson's Disease.

California uses 250 million pounds of pesticides annually (about one fourth of the U.S. total). *The incidence of Parkinson's Disease is higher in the counties where these chemicals are being used.*

Another study found that persons newly diagnosed with Parkinson's Disease (P.D.) who had high pesticide exposure in their homes were 70% more likely to have P.D. than a control test of persons without the disease. We think that NDF might help Parkinson's Disease(Chapter 32).

This exposure as a factor of civilized life makes it imperative that we take potent antioxidants daily to block the damaging effects of the free radicals we all are exposed to.

There are some natural substances that eliminate insects in a safe manner. Orange Guard, which is a water based extract of orange peels, kills all insects. This can be obtained from Orange Guard Inc., Carmel Valley, CA (www.orangeguard.com)

Neem oil products, diatomaceous earth and boric acid are safe alternatives to chemical insecticides. EcoSmart of Franklin, Tennessee has a line of natural insecticides, some using eugenol, the oil of cloves, and others using tree and plant essential oils that can be used for agricultural markets as well as homes. Contact them at 888-326-7233.

Problems With White Bread

Eating white bread has caused seizures in dogs, presumably because of the loss of nutrients, which occurs in the creation of white flour. The addition of vitamins, emulsifiers, and other ingredients makes white bread a *very artificial food*. White flour is treated with improvers when milled and then receives oxidizing agents, bleaches, chemical water that has been treated with alum, soda ash, copper sulfate and chlorine. Chemical leaveners may include sodium bicarbonate, alum, tartrates, phosphates, starch and cream of tartar.

Baking, using cake mixes, frozen dough, self rising flour, and processed foods, consumes 19 million kilograms of sodium aluminum phosphate (SAP) annually. The quantity of SAP averages 3 to 3.5% of each item baked. Additionally, 300,000 kg. of sodium aluminum sulfate is used in household baking powder, averaging 21 to 26% of the bulk of these products. There is a some suspicion that aluminum is the cause of Alzheimer's Disease (See Chapter 26 on Dementia in the Elderly).

How Does The Commercial Oil Industry Manufacture The Fats We Eat?

The natural soybean, cottonseed, sunflower seed, canola, and peanut seed is washed then crushed and heated to 248 degrees to break up the cell wall facilitating the extraction of the oil. Living enzymes are destroyed by temperature over 110 degrees.

The dead mash of cooked seeds is then forced through a giant press which exerts up to several tons per square inch of pressure. As the seeds are forced against the press the friction generated raises the temperature to 203 degrees F. If the manufacturing process stops here the oils can be sold as "cold pressed, natural, crude, or unrefined", usually getting premium prices in health food stores.

Authorities agree that the high temperature of this manufacturing process has caused deterioration of the fatty acids in the original seed. *These "cold pressed" oils seem dreadful to me but they are the highest quality oil currently available from U.S. manufacturers.*

A second manufacturing process that is also widely used involves putting a chemical solvent (often hexane, a petroleum derivative) into the crushed and cooked seed mash, which is heated to 149 degrees F. This solvent unavoidably taints the oil. These chemically - derived oils are often mixed with so-called "cold pressed" oils and sold as unrefined oils.

Because the manufacturers believe that the consumer wants clear, easily pouring, odorless, and tasteless oils even more processing is done. Natural oils have color ranging from pale yellow to gold to red. Each has it's own distinctive aroma and taste.

The Refining Process

The remainder of the commercially constructed oil proceeds through the refining process, which has 8 steps :

Degumming removes most of the remaining phophatides, which are essential for life. Lecithin, complex carbohydrates, proteins, gums, chlorophyll, calcium, magnesium, iron, and copper all get refined out.

Corrosive chemicals, usually sodium hydroxide (DRANO) or a mixture of sodium hydroxide and sodium carbonate, are placed into the oil which is agitated at a temperature of 167 degrees F. The remaining fatty acids in the sludge react with the caustic chemicals to form soaps, which are easily removed. Nearly all proteins, minerals, and phospholipids are gone by this stage, but there is still a faint yellow or red hue.

The pigments are *bleached out* using acid based clays at temperatures of 230 degrees F. The few fatty acids still remaining have now been converted into toxic peroxides. Beta carotene, an important cancer preventative, and chlorophyll along with most of the fatty acids disappear during this "bleaching".

Deodorizing is essential, as the gentle aroma of natural seed oil has been replaced by unappetizing chemical odors and tastes. This requires steam distillation at a high temperature (518 degrees) for one hour. This removes the last remains of Vitamin E but does get rid of the dangerous peroxides and some pesticides. *At this stage the essential fatty acids your body needs have been transformed into a completely foreign material.*

Synthetic chemical antioxidants are added to increase shelf life and a de-foaming agent is used. Because some persons refrigerate their oil, the oil is artificially cooled and filtered again to ensure clarity in cold temperature.

Hydrogenation: The fatty acid residue is then saturated with hydrogen under pressure at a temperature of 410 degrees F. Nickel, platinum or copper is used to catalyze this reaction, which goes on for 8 hours. The end product is *completely dead and will not spoil and tolerates heating without becoming toxic.* Chemically altered pieces of fatty acids remain, which may be harmful and there are still traces of the metal catalyst.

Partial Hydrogenation: By controlling the length of the hydrogenating process, the liquid oil can be changed into either a solid or a semisolid mass (margarine). This partially hydrogenated substance *is more dangerous to health than full hydrogenation because the oil molecules have been bombarded with hydrogen in an erratic manner, leaving a proliferation of strange substances that the body recognizes as harmful because they interfere with normal metabolism.*

Clever advertising has convinced us margarine is good because it has polyunsaturated fats. *However, these polyunsaturated fats are not the essential fatty acids the body desperately need, but chemically altered alien fats, which seem to play a major role in the causation of degenerative diseases. Many medical scientific experts feel that the body has adverse reactions to a trace amount of chemically altered foreign substances. The cumulative effects of regularly consuming a diet high in chemically altered fat is devastating.*

Margarines contain an average of 30% chemically altered fat (CAF). Vegetable oil contains 15% CAF. Commercial baked goods contain 35% CAF. Candies contain 40% CAF. Peanut butter has variable amounts of CAF, while french fries and potato chips contain 40%. The American public now consumes more than one *billion* pounds of hydrogenated oils annually. Go through a supermarket to see if you can find any products that do not contain hydrogenated fats and added sugar.

What you see in your supermarket labeled as corn, soy, safflower, and sunflower margarines and oils has nothing to do with corn, soybeans, safflower, and sunflower. *This material labeled as corn, soy, safflower, and sunflower is actually an artificial chemical substance that, in time, can be harmful to the human body.*

Food Irradiation

Companies that are stuck with radioactive waste material have a huge problem on their hands. These substances are dangerous and very expensive to dispose of. They have successfully persuaded the government to allow them to use these radioactive waste products to irradiate food.

The human body was not designed to metabolize food that has been transformed by radiation and there is a strong probability these new artificial foods will be just as harmful to health, or worse, than the synthetic transfats.

Research in the 1950's revealed *that animals who ate irradiated food developed premature death, an unusual form of cancer, reproductive failure, chromosomal abnormalities, liver damage, trouble gaining weight and vitamin deficiencies.*

Irradiation destroys vitamins, essential fatty acids and other nutrients. Radiation destroys 80% of the Vitamin A in eggs and 48% of the beta carotene in orange juice, but still is authorized by the FDA to be used in these foods.

The flavor, odor and texture of food is transformed. Pork become red; beef can smell like a wet dog and eggs can become colorless, runny and capable of ruining recipes. Whether protein after being injured by radiation will still be capable of functioning as building blocks for body protein is problematic.

More likely, the body will be damaged by efforts to dispose of artificial fats, carbohydrates and protein created by radiation (radiolytic products). These radiolytic products have not been studied for safety.

Irradiation will encourage even worse hygienic conditions in our slaughterhouses, where currently significant percentages of the meat from the cattle, pork and chickens have positive cultures for pathogenic bacteria.

Some irradiation plants may begin using caesium 137 which was left over from the production of nuclear weapons. This radioactive material is dangerous and unstable. In 1988 a leak of caesium 137 near Atlanta cost thirty million dollars to clean up.

Radiation does increase the shelf life of food which will enable the large food conglomerates to gain even more control over the production, distribution and selling of foods. *Learn to recognize the label for radiated products and refuse to buy them.*

The Grave Problems of the Meat Industry

When an industry falls into the hands of a few companies that are more interested in profits than the quality of their products, serious problems often appear. This is the current situation of the meat industry. Many dangerous substances are now found in U.S. beef. Among them are:

Pesticides

Nearly all meat has been contaminated with toxic chemicals that are applied to livestock and ingested from animal feed. Crops grown to be fed to life stock *have no limit to the quantity of pesticides that may be applied to the crops.* These chemicals accumulate in cattle so the quantity of pesticide from eating meat is greater than from eating plant foods.

Dioxin

Dioxin is a term applied to hundreds of chemicals that all have the quality of persisting in the environment. These substances are considered to be among the most toxic of all known poisons. They have been implicated in heart disease, endometriosis, falling sperm counts, rising numbers of testicular cancers and breast cancer.

They are often unintentional byproducts of industrial processes involving *chlorine*, such as waste incineration, manufacturing of chemicals and pesticides and the bleaching of pulp and paper. These were the primary components of "Agent Orange" and were also found in the Love Canal clean up.

The US Environmental Protection Agency report that 95% of human exposure is from eating beef, pork, chicken, milk, fish and eggs. Dioxins are water phobic, so that if present in a lake or river, they move into the fish.

Fats

There has been a striking change in the character of meat in the past 50 years. Meat has gone from being a good food that accumulated essential fatty acids and conjugated linoleic acid from grazing, into a food that is bad for health. Feed-lot raised cattle are fed sorghum, a high sugar waste product of sugar mills and grain which helps them gain weight rapidly. These feed-lot cattle produce stearic acid fat which, when eaten by humans, causes elevation of cholesterol and LDL (bad) cholesterol.

Chemical pesticides become concentrated in fat tissue. In 1991, 36 nations studied the consumption of animal and dairy fat. They discovered a direct correlation between the quantity of these fats consumed and the development of cancer of the prostate, colon, lung and breast. This can be reversed by eating organic beef and dairy products (no hormones, pesticides or antibiotics).

Antibiotics

Meat producing animals are routinely given antibiotics to speed up their growth. This means that penicillin, tetracycline and other antibiotics that are used in treating human disease are being given to healthy cattle. This has become a leading cause for antibiotic resistant bacteria that are no longer easy to eliminate in human diseases. Perhaps as much as 75% of all antibiotic usage in the US *is in healthy animals.*

Because of the problem of antibiotic resistance, Europe now restricts livestock antibiotic usage to 4 antibiotics which are excluded from being used in treating human illnesses. The problems of antibiotic and hormone contamination of meat has led Europe to refuse importation of US meat.

Since 1995 the FDA has permitted the use of implanted hormones in cattle. These hormones include estradiol, progesterone, norgestomet, testosterone and the synthetic anabolic steroids, seranol and trenbolone. These estrogens given to cattle are widely recognized as contributing to the estrogen dominance of humans. *The former director of endocrinology at the National Cancer Institute, Dr. Ray Harris, warned in the 1980's that this disturbance in the hormonal balance was likely to precipitate problems with cancer.* Estradiol, the hormone most commonly used to fatten cattle, is a potent cancer-causing estrogen. Confidential industry reports reveal the presence of high hormone residues in meat. In this manner, the US population is consuming, without warning or labeling, hormones from meat.

A USDA survey of 32 large feed-lots revealed that nearly 50% had visible illegal hormone muscle implants, instead of the proper location in the ear. This could result in very high hormone levels in meat.   Since the 1950's, breast cancer has increased by 55%, testicular cancer by 120%, prostrate cancer by 190%. Some of this increase must be related to disturbed hormonal balance in humans resulting from hormonal implants in cattle.

Growth Hormones

Monsanto developed a recombinant Bovine Growth Hormone called Posilic which increases milk production by 20% This extra milk production was associated with great stress to the cows as it interfered with reproduction, caused mastitis requiring more antibiotics and led to premature death in the animals. To overcome these new problems the agricultural industry began to feed the dairy cows a high protein diet.

These proteins were obtained form diseased cows (downer cows), live stock that died of old age, disease or accidents, wasted inedible meat from slaughterhouses and supermarkets, deceased zoo animals, euthanized pets and road kill.

This rendering of disposable animal remains has grown into a 3 billion dollar industry. The bad decision to turn cows into cannibals has been compounded by another bad decision to feed diseased contaminated protein to cows. One would have assumed that shortening the life span of a milk producing cow would have been enough reason to terminate the use of bovine growth hormones, but apparently the ability to use dead cows in an economic manner caused the use of growth hormone to continue.

For many years it has been known that growth hormone extracted from dead cows when injected into living animals would increase milk production. In humans extracted growth hormones from cadavers was use to produce growth in hypopituitary dwarfs. This had to be terminated when it was discovered that 14 of the 8000 persons treated died of Creutzfeld-Jacob disease. This illness is caused by a very small infectious particle called a prion, which must have been contained in the growth home injected into the dwarfs. These particles are too small to be seen by an electron microscope and cannot be cultured. Recombinant growth hormone is how used for this condition.

Mad Cow Disease (BSE) and Creutzfeld-Jacob Disease

Mad Cow Disease (BSE) began to appear in Great Britain in 1980. This disease has similar pathology to Creutzfeld-Jacob Disease (CJD) found in humans. In BSE the brain takes on a spongy appearance, as it is full of holes. Similar spongy appearing brain tissues can be found in many animal disease. Some of these diseases appear to be caused by infectious particles called prions.

In 1997 the FDA banned the feeding of cattle parts to cattle but cattle were still permitted to eat horses and pig protein. Pigs eating scrapie (prion) infected sheep could still infect cows with BSE.

What Should Beef Lovers Do?

One solution is to become a vegetarian. The other is to find a cattle rancher who will grow cattle by grazing and who refused to implant hormones and use antibiotics or pesticide contaminated feed. Such a rancher deserves to be paid a premium price for his meat which is safe to eat. This meat has high levels of the desired Omega 3 fatty acids and 5 times more of healthy conjugated linoleic acid than feedlot cattle.

My guess is that struggling cattle ranchers might be delighted to find a ready market for their beef at higher prices. Ask at your local health food store. Local people who are health conscious may know local sources. Check around and you may be pleasantly surprised to find good, safe beef available from small producers. A final solution could be to buy beef imported from Argentina. Argentine beef is grazed and is superb.

Chapter 3

Immune Illnesses

Thymic Extract

Thymic extract is the story of Dr. Carlos Burgstiner of Georgia. Dr. Burgstiner was an Obstetrician Gynecologist who developed a Hepatitis B infection. The possible transmission of this virus to a patient prevented him from doing surgery.

In his search to become well he began to take thymic extract combined with vitamins. Six weeks later his blood test for Hepatitis B became negative *after seven years of illness*. This combination of ingredients had corrected a problem in his immune systems ability to fight off the hepatitis virus.

By 1998 treatment with this compound led to the following results:

- 84 cases of Hepatitis B arrested

- 34 cases of Hepatitis C arrested

- 28 cases of Rheumatoid Arthritis arrested

- 12 cases of Systemic Lupus Erythematosus arrested

- 10 cases of Multiple Sclerosis arrested

- 12 cases of Psoriasis arrested

Hepatitis C is a very serious illness which kills many people. Patients with Hepatitis C taking thymic extract have improved and had their hepatitis C blood tests revert to normal.

HIV Infection

HIV infection is an illness resulting in the complete destruction of the immune system. Many persons with HIV are taking thymic extract and appear to have stabilized.

Thymic Extract can be obtained from Preventative Therapeutics 800 556 5530 and from *Natural Health Team.* 800-4162806

Dimethyl Glycine (DMG)

Research studies have shown that DMG can have a dramatic effect on the immune system. This ability is called immune modulation, which means that this substance can restore or increase the response of the immune system.

Russian researchers have claimed that DMG could restore the immune system in persons whose immune system had been destroyed by full body radiation. The substance has been found to be completely safe.

Who might benefit from this therapy?

- Patients with HIV infection

- Persons exposed to radiation poisoning.

- The chronically ill child

- Patients who have been on radiation and chemotherapy, which has nearly destroyed the immune system

- Patients who undergo organ transplants

Prior to the transplant the patient is given treatments to destroy the immune system so there is less chance for the transplant to be rejected. When the period of probable rejection has passed, DMG could prove valuable.

Hazards Of Root Canal Surgery

Root canal operations are among the most common in dentistry, with millions being done every year. This operation is performed in an attempt to save a tooth that has experienced damage to the dentin and pulp from a caries infection.

In this operation, the pulp is removed and a packing is placed in the cavity to try to sterilize the area. Dr. Weston Price, a brilliant dental researcher, found that it was impossible to sterilize the root canal cavity. Obviously any bacteria that remained were free to multiply and potentially could construct an abscess in the canal cavity.

Dr. Price persuaded a patient who had developed a wheel chair confining arthritis after having root canal surgery that she needed to have the root canal tooth removed.

He then placed the extracted tooth under the skin of a rabbit. Within two days the rabbit had developed a disabling arthritis.

The woman made a complete recovery. Dr. Price confirmed these results many times, but his research was ignored until Dr. George Meining published his break-through book on this subject, *Root Canal Surgery Cover-Up Exposed.*

Dr. Weston Price spent 25 years studying the direct relationship between the performance of root canal surgery and the *subsequent* development of a degenerative health problem (heart disease, arthritis, kidney disease, bacteremia, endocarditis, phlebitis, anemia, leukopenia, back, neck and shoulder pain, neuritis, etc.) .

This information raises important questions. Should the root canal tooth be removed?

There would not appear to be any reason to do this unless the person had developed an illness that could be related to the dental abscess.

Should Root Canals Be Done?

Certainly any person with an occult immune problem, (early HIV, early leukemia, diabetes, elderly, cancer victims) should probably avoid this operation. Even young healthy people with a presumably normal immune system can have this surgery and become critically ill after the operation. (See Dr. Atkin's case below)

Should teeth with existing root canals be removed? Certainly they should, if there is any possible link to a subsequent illness the patient develops. *I can see a problem. When you are elderly, is anyone going to connect the root canal you had thirty years ago with the current degenerative illness?*

Most MDs do not inquire about root canals in their inventory of past illness. Very few physicians are aware that root canal surgery can be responsible for the subsequent development of a chronic degenerative process.

Dr. Robert Atkins had a patient who knew of the danger of root canals. This woman had an 11 year old child as a neighbor. The child had a root canal three days earlier and had slipped into a coma and was "going fast".

When this information was given to his patient, the patient insisted that the MD contact Dr. Atkins. After much arguing with several of those caring for her, an intelligent Maxillary-facial surgeon asked the obvious question, *"What do we have to lose?" Within an hour after the removal of the root canal tooth, the child was awake and up and walking. This case does illustrate that a presumably healthy young person can face possibly deadly consequences from root canal surgery* .

Any surgical procedure that creates a permanent abscess in the body must be considered potentially dangerous. Better techniques for performing this operation are badly needed.

Elderberry

(See Chapter 28 on resistant Bacteria, Candida and Viruses)

Immunocal

Immunocal is a milk-serum- protein concentrate that raises cellular glutathione levels. Glutathione is a powerful free radical scavenger. Sick people are deficient in glutathione (GTH). GTH is composed of three amino acids glutamine, cysteine, and glycine. Cysteine is lacking in most diets whereas the other two aminoacids are readily available. Immunocal provides the needed cysteine and thus may be an effective way to boost cellular GTH levels.

Fibromyalgia

Fibromyalgia is a common condition characterized by severe painful areas in the body, insomnia, and depression. (This will be discussed in more detail in Chapter 6 Rheumatoid Arthritis.) Immunocal has brought prompt relief to several persons with fibromyalgia, suggesting that GTH deficiency might be playing a role in the causation of this syndrome.

Cataracts

A patient was diagnosed with early full lens cataracts. Four months later, he began to take Immunocal, which was followed by dissolution of his cataracts. Cataracts are known to be deficient in Glutathione. Immunocal can be purchased from Lifestar Millenium 800-8587477

Sterinol

Researchers in South Africa have developed this product after 20 years of study. This substance helps situations in which the immune response is underactive, such as cancer and AIDS. However, it also benefits conditions in which the immune system is overactive, attacking healthy tissue (rheumatoid arthritis, diabetes).

The immune system protects us from outside bacteria, viruses, and parasites, but also needs to destroy abnormal cancer cells and toxins that were eaten or breathed.

Anything that the immune system does not recognize as a friend, (the body's own tissue or helpful bacteria and nutrients) is tagged to be removed. An out of control immune system that attacks friendly tissue can be just as dangerous as one that permits cancer cells to multiply.

A specific T cell (TH 1) produces interleukin-2, which increases the immune response to bacteria, viruses, and cancer cells. When an infection is defeated, this same Th 1 stops producing antibodies. If there are not enough Th 1 cells, there are insufficient Natural Killer Lymphocytes produced and infections and cancer gain ground.

A different T cell named Th 2 produces interleukin 4, 6, and 10. These three interleukins stimulate the inflammatory reaction and allergic responses. *If there is too much Th 2 activity, there will be excessive antibody production which leads to worsening of allergic problems and appearance of autoimmune illnesses, where the body attacks its own tissues..*

Sterinol appears to increase killer lymphocyte activity and Th1, while stopping the undesirable Th 2 action.

Sterinol is made from soy and pine. All plants contain fat molecules called sterols. In nature these sterols are always accompanied by molecules called sterolins. The correct ratio of sterols to sterolins is needed for an immune enhancing effect. Sterolins are easily destroyed by processing and the key to this therapy was finding a way to preserve the sterolin through the extraction process. Dr. Patrick Bouic was the lead researcher. Sterinol has been used for many years in Germany as *Harzol*.

Clinical Results

Rheumatoid Arthritis

This illness is an autoimmune problem resulting from inadequate Th 1 activity, which permits Th 2 to produce antibodies that attack the joints.

One patient illustrates the capability of sterinol treatment. This woman was 32 years old when she contracted a severe form of RA, which had disabling arthritis, and golf ball sized lumps on her elbows. These lumps are seen only in severe cases of RA. She started Sterinol after cortisone had failed to help her. After 4 months, the pain subsided and she was able to stop cortisone. *She is now well and has been off sterinol for 25 years.*

Type 1 Diabetes (Insulin Needing)

There is evidence that this condition is related to antibodies that attack the pancreatic islet cells. Insulin treatment has been able to be decreased in patients taking sterolin. Physician guidance regarding insulin dosage is a necessity.

HIV: In a study of 323 HIV patients, those taking sterinol had steady helper T cell levels, while those not receiving sterinol saw helper T cells steadily decline.

Hepatitis C: Patients with this disorder usually see rapid return of liver enzyme tests to normal after starting sterinol.

Benign Prostatic Hypertrophy: Two hundred patients received sterinol or a placebo. Those getting sterinol noted improved urine flow and decrease in symptoms, without side effects.

Sterinol is also reported to benefit patients with lupus, multiple sclerosis, Parkinson's Disease, Crohn's Disease, celiac disease, psoriasis, scleroderma, asthma, hives, eczema, herpes, shingles, tuberculosis, chronic fatigue syndrome, ulcerative colitis, fibromyalgia, rheumatic fever, and irritable bowel syndrome.

Much more information about Sterinol can be found in Dr. Bouic's book *The Immune System Cure* (Prentice Hall 1999),

Sterinol can be purchased from Advanced Nutritional Products 888-436 7200 and from our *Natural Health Team* 800-4162806.

Soil Based Organisms: This substance has significant benefits to the immune system and will be discussed in depth in Chapter 17 Gastrointestinal Disease.

Padma Therapy For Immune Disorders

Padma has the ability to restore balance to the immune system in the same way Sterinol does. Patients with Hepatitis B and other viral hepatitis appear to be injured by the body's immune cells attacking the liver cells invaded by the virus.

After treating 126 adults and 52 children with chronic Hepatitus B with Padma, nearly all patients exhibited significant improvement. In 15% of cases the Hepatitus was healed. In 90% blood chemistry was returned to normal. All patients received 2 tablets of Padma three times daily and

1000mg. of gamma linoleic acid daily.

Padma also appears to protect the liver from alcohol injury.

Patients with HIV having Aids –related complex lymphoadenopathy and Kaposi's Sarcoma all stabilized with Padma therapy.

Chapter 4

Heart Diseases

The proper diet for patients with angina and heart attacks to follow has been a source of controversy. The two parts of the world that have the lowest incidence of arteriosclerotic heart disease are the island of Crete and the Japanese island of Kohama. People in both these places eat a diet that is high in linolenic acid, an *essential* fatty acid. The Cretans get their linolenic acid from walnuts and purslane, whereas the Japanese islanders are getting their linolenic acid from soybeans and canola oil (rapeseed oil).

Researchers in France followed 605 patients after a first heart attack, with one half receiving the American Heart Association Diet (low cholesterol) and the other half receiving the Cretan Diet (lots of whole grains, roots, and green vegetables, fish, daily fruit, chicken and olive oil). The study was terminated at 27 months and all patients were switched to the Cretan diet because of dramatic benefits from this diet (see chart)

	American Heart Association Diet	Mediterranean Diet
Total # of Heart Attacks	33	8
Deaths from Heart attacks	16	3
Sudden Death	8	0

Linolenic acid has two desirable qualities. It makes blood less likely to clot and prevents ventricular arrhythmias. Note the 8 sudden deaths in the AHA diet and the absence of sudden death in the Cretan diet.

Sudden death is caused by an electrical gradient being established between an area of well oxygenated heart muscle and an adjacent area of poorly oxygenated heart muscle. This gradient often permits ventricular fibrillation to occur. This is a condition where purposeless, small, feeble muscle contractions move no blood and cause instant death. This is seen often in smokers, where the nicotine constricts a coronary artery so much a gradient is created leading to ventricular fibrillation. *When smokers quit cigarettes their incidence of sudden death instantly returns to the same as a nonsmoker.*

Tragically, in approximately 35% of individuals, the presence of serious coronary artery arteriosclerosis is confirmed only by the occurrence of sudden death.

Linolenic acid is found mainly in seeds (flax, hemp, soybean, walnut, pumpkin), as it is easily destroyed by light, air, and heat. *By the end of 27 months, the blood linolenic acid levels in the French patients had reached the same range as those seen in Crete.*

Hypertension

Hypertension afflicts about 15% of the U.S. populace. This is a very serious condition because long standing increased pressure against the lining wall of arteries creates injury to the lining (endothelium) in which arteriosclerotic plaques are prone to develop. Heart attacks are much more frequent in hypertensive patients than persons with normal blood pressure.

Untreated or poorly controlled high blood pressure is often complicated by enlargement of the heart. Over time the workload on the heart becomes such a burden that the heart becomes larger and may eventually fail to pump blood effectively, leading to fluid retention (congestive heart failure).

In addition, the extra pressure against arteries in the brain makes them more likely to rupture causing bleeding into brain substance (cerebral hemorrhage), which is often fatal.

Lowering blood pressure with either pharmaceutical or natural health treatments will significantly decrease the risk of hypertension.

Actuarial studies of blood pressure by insurance companies show that the mean blood pressure is directly correlated with survival. These studies have even shown that persons whose blood pressure is "normal" at 135/85 do not survive as well as those whose blood pressure is 125/75. This raises an interesting question: what is normal blood pressure and should therapy of high blood pressure be more vigorous?

The pharmaceutical companies have created a large number of drugs that are effective at lowering blood pressure. These drugs uniformly have a problem with side effects, some of which can be serious.

Can blood pressure be brought to normal by *natural* treatments?

The answer is yes.

Magnesium

The cornerstone of natural therapy for hypertension is magnesium, which can be given as oxide, aspartate, or a mixture of both. Magnesium relaxes the musculature in the walls of the arteries, permitting the artery to widen and the blood within the artery then exerts less pressure against the wall of the artery (Vasodilatation). This results in lower blood pressure until the effect of the magnesium wears off.

Because the action of magnesium is a physiologic effect of the magnesium ion on arterioles *it will work for all persons.* Some pharmaceutical drugs used in treatment of hypertension vary in effectiveness depending on age, sex, Afro-American, Oriental, and other subgroups. Afro-Americans often respond better to diuretic therapy than Caucasians.

The magnesium ion also acts as a stimulant to the gastrointestinal tract, which means that high magnesium doses may be associated with frequent bowel movements.

This action of magnesium in the body as a vasodilator has long been used in obstetrics to lower the blood pressure in eclampsia.

Intravenous magnesium given during a heart attack improves the survival rate, probably by preventing extra ventricular heartbeats, which can lead to dangerous heart rhythms.

The maintenance dose for blood pressure control needs to be 1000 mg. or more daily.

Another agent of great importance in bringing the blood pressure down and keeping it down is omega 3 fatty acids in the form of flax oil.

Flax Oil

In a paper from The American Journal of Clinical Nutrition vol. 44: Sept. 1986 Dr. E. M. Berry reported that a *1% increase in dietary linolenic acid was associated with a healthy decrease in blood pressure*. Linolenic acid is only one eighth the quantity of linoleic acid in the usual diet but it has a disproportionately large effect on blood pressure, probably because of its beneficial influence on prostaglandin secretion by the kidney. The linolenic acid leads to the production of *prostaglandins that lower blood pressure*.

This flax can be obtained as 2 tablespoons of flax oil or 4 tablespoons of ground flaxseed taken daily.

Coenzyme Q10 (Co Q10)

Co Q10 has been found to be of value in treating inflammatory injury (myocarditis) to the heart from viral infections and other causes. There also is a beneficial effect in lowering blood pressure. The daily doses needed vary between 180 mg. and 360 mg.

Coenzyme Q10 was given to 109 cardiology patients who had hypertension for at least one year. They were given an average dose of 225 mg. daily. Blood tests were used to insure that the blood level of Co Q10 was over 2.0 mcg/ml.

Fifty one per cent of these patients were able to discontinue between one and three of their usual blood pressure medicines by four and one half months into the study. The thickness of the heart muscle in the left side of the heart was found to exhibit a beneficial decrease and the main chamber of the heart (left ventricle) showed improved function in the 9.4% of patients who had an echocardiogram before and after the study.

Be sure your blood pressure is being monitored regularly, *as not all patients respond to Co Q10*. If there is no benefit in two months consider trying a different treatment.

Another valuable property of CoQ10 is its great benefit in the condition diastolic dysfunction. In the past ten years two forms of heart failure have been delineated (systolic and diastolic). Systolic heart failure is widely recognized in the medical profession. In this state the heart fails to pump blood adequately, resulting in enlargment of the heart with fluid collecting in the lungs, liver, gastrointestinal tract and extremities.

In the diastolic form of heart failure trouble develops as the left side of the heart fills with blood. This has incorrectly been assumed to be a period of rest for the heart as it fills with blood. Actually the energy needed to stretch so the extra blood can be accommodated in the left ventricle is greater than the energy need to pump blood out of the left ventricle.

There is no problem with the heart's pumping action, but the failed filling of the heart leads to shortness of breath and fatigue. The echocardigram confirms the diagnosis.

Many patients with diastolic heart failure are women with a long history of high blood pressure. Therapy with the nutrient CoQ10 effectively lowers blood pressure and improves diastolic function of the heart with disappearance of shortness of breath and fatigue. The dosage needed may vary from from 200 mg to 300 mg. daily, in divided doses.

There are no known harmful side effects. Co Q10 is readily available at most health food stores. The gel form is believed to be better absorbed.

L-Arginine

This natural element lowers blood pressure by 20 mm. in two weeks. The dose can be increased to 6 grams daily in divided doses.

This can be purchased in health food stores and from *Natural Health Team*.

Olive Leaf Extract

Olive leaf extract has enabled patients with hypertension to decrease or eliminate blood pressure medicines. The dose is 500 mg. three times daily. The effect of olive leaf takes two weeks to develop and the blood pressure falls by 5 to 15 mm. Systolic and 5 to 8 mm. Diastolic.

Olive leaf extract can be purchased from Nature's Distributors 800-624 7114.

Dietary Changes

Dr. John McDougall of the St. Helena Clinic has seen hundreds of patients with high blood pressure experience falls in their blood pressure after being started on a vegetarian diet.

This is well demonstrated by the example of Sam, who was on three drugs for hypertension when he entered the St. Helena Clinic. His blood pressure was 158/104 on admission. The following day it had fallen to 148/90. By the 9th day his blood pressure was *110/70 and he was off all medicine.*

Intake of magnesium, calcium, and potassium from food may protect against the development of high blood pressure and may be very beneficial in lowering blood pressure in those who have elevated blood pressure. The foods that help are fresh fruit, vegetables and high fiber low fat foods (whole grains).

Steady heavy intake of alcohol raises the blood pressure, and giving up alcohol or curtailing alcohol intake may be very helpful in lowering the blood pressure.

If you are not ready for a vegetarian diet, the Mediterranean diet should also help as it contains far less animal fat and increases the fruit and vegetable content compared to the standard U. S. diet.

Flaxseed

Ingestion of flaxseed on a daily basis lowers blood pressure by causing increased output of beneficial prostaglandins from the kidney, which lower blood pressure.

Exertion

Regular physical exertion lowers the blood pressure. The mechanism which accomplishes this may be improved oxygenation of the kidney, which is associated with the release of blood pressure lowering prostaglandins.

Weight Loss

Physicians have long known that weight loss lowers blood pressure.

Even slight weight loss brings improvement. If a patient is able to lose 20 to 25 pounds *the blood pressure often returns to normal.*

Essential Oils

In 1920 a French cosmetic chemist named Rene-Maurice Gattefosse sustained severe burns on an arm in a laboratory accident. He plunged his arm into a vessel that he believed contained water. The vessel actually contained pure lavender oil. Much to his surprise the pain ceased in a few moments and continued application of the lavender oil permitted *healing without scarring.*

In World War 2 his colleague, Dr. Jean Valnet, was stationed in China treating battlefield casualties. When they began running out of antibiotics Dr. Valnet began to use essential oils. These oils exerted powerful healing effects and saved many lives even some patients who probably would have perished had antibiotics been available.

In the 17th century during the Black Plague a band of thieves robbed the deceased without becoming ill. They were apothecaries and had rubbed essential oils on their skin daily which protected them from this plague.

The city of Bucklersbury, England was spared from the plague. This city was the center for the European lavender trade. The oil of lavender has immune stimulating and antimicrobial properties that rival and even surpass modem antiseptic chemicals and antibiotics.

What Are Essential Oils?

Essential oils are the subtle, volatile liquids, or resins from plants, shrubs, flowers, trees, roots, bushes, and seeds. They give plants and trees characteristic odors such as rose, cedar or pine. There are 30,000 known aromatic molecules and multitudes have yet to be discovered.

The essential oils are the regenerating and oxygenating defense properties of plants. These oxygenating molecules transport nutrients and other powerful chemicals to the plant cells which brings life to the plants, destroys infections, aids growth, fights off infestations, and stimulates healing. They are to plants what blood is to the human body.

Three primary elements are found in all essential oils (hydrogen, carbon and oxygen). These oils contain other powerful chemicals including alcohols, phenols, esters, ethers, oxides, coumarins, terpinols, ketones and aldehydes.

The oils are manufactured in the plant in specialized structures including secretory cells, glands, glandular hairs and resin ducts. In a process similar to photosynthesis plants create essential oils by trapping and transmuting light and energy. The secretory cells that produce the volatile oils trap the photoelectromagnetic energy of the sun and, with the help of glucose, convert it into biochemical energy in the form of aromatic molecules. This process creates some of the most powerful natural healing elements known to man. These oils penetrate cell walls and transport oxygen, nutrients and other vital chemicals into each cell. They constitute the life force of the plant.

Some of the chief chemicals in the essential oils include:

- *Aldehydes*: The aldehydes have anti-infectious, anti-inflammatory, antiseptic, calming and sedative properties. They include lemongrass, melissa, citronella, and citral.

- *Phenols*: These are deadly for bacteria. They contain oxygenating molecules and are powerful antioxidants. These include thymol, eugenol, and carvacrol which has anti-cancer properties.

- *Alcohols*: These are strongly anti-bacterial and anti-viral. The sequiterpenol molecules in this group have anti-inflammatory and immune stimulating properties. They increase the oxygenation of the pineal and pituitary glands.

- *Terpenes*: These inhibit the accumulation of toxins in the body and help the liver and kidneys eliminate toxins. They have antiseptic, stimulating, antiinflammatory, antiviral, antibacterial, analgesic, antispasmodic and sedative qualities.

- *Ketones*: These are known to stimulate cell regeneration and promote the formation of tissue. Because they help dissolve and discharge mucous they benefit asthma, colds, and influenza.

- *Esters*: These are the product of alcohol reacting with an acid. They have a relaxing soothing effect in the body. They also are anti-spasmodic and are quite effective against fungi.

One of the principle characteristics of essential oils (EO) is their containment of a multitude of powerful oxygenating molecules. This explains why EO applied to the skin or when inhaled (aromatherapy) dramatically increases cellular oxygenation.

When applied to the skin EO penetrates every cell in the body within 21 minutes. They even go into fingernails and toenails to attack fungi. Dried herbs require 13 to 23 hours to reach therapeutic levels in the cells after ingestion.

Because essential oils are very concentrated most of them are at least *50 times more potent than the herbs they are derived from*. The oils contain nearly all the healing nutrients, oxygenating molecules, amino acid precursors, coenzyme A factors, trace minerals, enzymes, vitamins, and hormones found in the plant. When herbs are cut and dehydrated for human treatment they can lose up to 90% of the healing nutrients contained within as well as much of the oxygen molecules.

This concentrated effect has caused many physicians to consider essential oils to actually be medicine. The EO from thyme destroys anthrax bacillus, typhoid bacillus, glanders bacillus, diptheria bacillus, meningococcus and tuberculosis bacilli.

Professor Griffon, Director of the French Police Toxicology Laboratory, studied the purifying effect of a blend of aerosolized pine, thyme, peppermint, lavender, rosemary and cloves on harmful bacteria in the air. Petri dishes were allowed to stand for 24 hours at a level 15 cm. above the floor. These dishes grew 210 different colonies of bacteria and molds. Within 15 minutes after spraying the room with the EO aerosol mixture only 14 of the original 210 were still alive. *All colonies of molds and bacteria were dead in 30 minutes.*

Dr. Valnet recommends "The administration of essential oils by fine aerosol spray should be common practice in sick rooms, operating rooms, and clinics". Dr. Valnet points out that pathogenic organisms (bacteria and viruses) do not become resistant to essential oils which means that the problems of resistant bacteria will not appear after repeated exposure to essential oils. Furthermore, essential oils are harmless to human tissue unlike chemical antiseptics.

Another great benefit is that many essential oils have strong anti-viral properties whereas antibiotics have no effect on viruses.

Non-healing incisions containing cancer tissue can be successfully treated with EO because these essences increase blood supply which encourages healing and damages malignant tissue which can not tolerate tissue oxygen.

Quick healing occurs in all nonhealing ulcers with EO usage and many chronic dermatitis problems also respond favorably to topical EO.

At this point in time essential oils have been shown to benefit by oxygenating, stimulating the immune response, rejuvenating tissue, increasing mineralization, anti-microbial effects, anti viral effects, antisepsis, anti-neuritic, anti-inflammatory, anti-fungal, antioxidant, anti-toxin, anti-venom qualities, promoting sleep and improving mood.

Frequencies Of Essential Oils

To understand essential oils better it is important to be aware of frequency. Frequency is the measurable rate of electrical energy flow between any two points. The human body has an electrical frequency and considerable information about an individual's health can be ascertained from their electrical frequency. (Dr. Robert 0. Becker's book The Body Electric).

In 1992 a pioneering scientist and researcher, Bruce Taino, built a bio-frequency monitor. This has shown that the average frequency of the human body during the day varies from 62 to 72 Hz. When this frequency drops substantially, *it is a clear indication that the immune system has been compromised.* When the frequency goes down to *58* Hz, colds and flu may appear. At 55hz, diseases indicative of immune compromise (Candida fungus) may appear. At 52 Hz, Epstein Barr and chronic fatigue syndrom may begin and at 42 Hz, cancer can occur.

Research has shown that when substances with low frequencies (junk food, synthetic drugs, poor quality vitamin and mineral supplements) come into contact with the human body the electrical frequency is rapidly pulled down to substandard levels creating a climate where disease and illness begin to flourish.

Processed and canned foods have a frequency of *zero.* These denatured foods represent the vast majority of American diet. Fresh produce has a frequency up to 15Hz. Dry herbs range from 12 to 22 Hz. Fresh herbs vary from 20 to 27 Hz. These can help the body maintain it's proper high electrical frequency.

When substances of higher frequency come in contact with disease causing organisms of a lower frequency the disease causing organisms are destroyed. Bruce Taino has recently demonstrated that the frequencies of essential oils range from 52 Hz to a whopping 320 Hz, depending on which oil was being studied. The essential oils have the highest frequencies of any substances known to man.

When used on the human body EO have the ability to raise the body's electrical frequency to high levels which creates an environment that facilitates the reduction of low frequency organisms such as bacteria, viruses, and fungi.

Dr. Valnet has recently discovered that the electrical constituents of the essential oil clove is opposed to cancer and viral diseases. *The essential oils clove, oregano, and cinnamon have the ability to prevent any pathogenic microorganism from surviving. At the same time they have no adverse effect on normal bacteria.*

How Can Essential Oils Be Used?

The two most popular ways to use essential oils are by diffusion into the air (aromatherapy) and direct application to the skin. Dr. Valnet states that whether inhaled or applied to the skin the essential oils have the same therapeutic effect. D. Gary Young points out that the body's response time to inhaled EO can be as quick as *one to three seconds.*

When inhaled odor particles travel up the nose and are trapped in the olfactory membranes. The olfactory nerves receive the vaporized oil particles and carry them along the nerve fiber to the olfactory bulb. While traveling the oils molecules trigger millions of nerve impulses that get dispatched to various parts of the body. Nerve impulses from the olfactory bulb go to the gustatory center (where the sensation of taste is perceived), the amygdala (where emotional memories are stored), and other parts of the limbic system where blood pressure, breathing, memory, stress levels, and hormone balance are controlled.

Smell is the only one of the five senses which is linked to the limbic lobe of the brain (emotional control center) which is the origin of anxiety, depression, fear, anger, and joy.

EO diffused in a home or office purifies the air by removing toxins, metallic particles, and other debris. They increase the oxygen content of the air, and boost levels of ozone, and negative ions that can inhibit the reproduction of airborne pathogens. As the oil particles disperse in a room they rapidly kill all harmful bacteria, viruses, molds, and fungi that they contact.

There are three ways to diffuse the oil in a room. In hot weather put a few drops on a kleenex near the air vent of a fan or air conditioner. The air blowing on this circulates the oil particles throughout the house.

The most used technique is to buy a diffuser which sprays an ultrafine mist into the air. These millions of particles are so fine they hang in the air for hours and become spread into every room by the normal circulation that follows walking.

Another favored way to diffuse involves using a mister of 4 to 6 ounces of the type used to spray house plants. Fill the mister with water and add 15 to 20 drops of essential oil. You can then walk through the house misting each room as you go.

All methods of diffusion are followed by immediate benefits. Using the oils in the room of a sick person who has flu or a cold will shorten the illness duration by *50%* or more.

Simply smelling the essential oil lavender from the bottle will terminate a stubborn sinus headache in 60 to 90 seconds. Smelling the oil of eucalyptus opens nasal passages and sinuses after several minutes. Smelling the EO peppermint for several minutes usually completely eliminates acid indigestion and heartburn. The EO birch or helichrysm often completely clears knee or joint pain when applied to the area. Both these oils contain anti-inflammatory and analgesic constituents as well as the usual oxygenating, immune boosting, and anti-microbial properties.

Other essential oils(rose, lavender, and ylang ylang) when rubbed up and down the spine at bedtime calm, relax, and usually result in a restful night of sleep.

Do not laugh but one of the best areas to place EO is specific areas on the soles of the feet. Within 21 minutes every cell of the body will have been penetrated by the oil regardless of where the oil was applied. The oxygen and micronutrients go right along into the cells in an extrordinarily efficient manner unmatched by any other product.

Unfortunately not all essential oils are the same. Most of the essential oils on the market are perfumer's grade which sell in health food stores and by discount mail order firms. These are overprocessed, chemical laden, highly adulterated and denatured products that are really cheap perfume made from odorous plants. They have little or none of the beneficial therapeutic qualities of *pure* essential oils.

Pure, unadulterated therapeutic essential oil is extremely difficult to locate and often very expensive. The reason for this is that it may take 500 to 2000 pounds of raw plant material to produce a single pound of pure essential oil. This pound of essential oil may cost from $1000 to $15,000 depending on the amount of plant needed and the difficulty of extraction.

The purity and therapeutic efficacy of the essential oil can also be greatly effected by the location the plants are grown in, the climate the plants are grown in, the growing procedures used, and the extraction procedures used. These plants must be organically grown in the right location, and at precisely the right climate. Harvesting often needs to be done by hand to avoid injuring the plant and it's delicate oil. The harvesting must be done at precisely the right time *when the oils in the plant are at peak potency.*

It is critical that the oils must be extracted by steam distillation at low pressure and low heat as all other methods (high heat and chemical extraction) rob the oils of their vitality. *These control factors are mandatory if the plant is to be sold as pure therapeutic quality.*

The only firm in the United States that is a major producer of essential oils and meets these quality standards is Young Living Essential Oils founded by Dr. Gary Young. Mr. Young has had extensive experience with essential oils in Europe and Egypt prior to starting his company. His farm in Idaho is the largest acreage of lavender in the U.S. and he was the first in North America to grow organic plants for distillation of essential oils. Some of his oils are imported from special farms in France, Egypt, Inner Mongolia, and China where the best locations and growing climates were located. Young carries 54 different kinds of pure essential oils and 45 different blends of pure therapeutic quality oils.

Their introductory kit contains three bottles of the most important and powerful essential healing oils (peppermint, lemon, and lavender) along with four bottles of blended essential oils. These are:

1. Lavender — This is used worldwide for healing severe burns, cuts, leg ulcers, bruises, and skin irritations. There is wide acceptance of lavender for headache reduction, insomnia, premenstrual syndrome, and stress. It kills staphlococcus, typhoid, diptheria, tuberculosis, pneumococci, hemolytic streptococci, and many other pathogens. It also has anti-venom properties.

2. Lemon — This oil is known to improve leukocyte formation and increase lymphocyte function which helps the immune system. It kills on contact meningococci, typhus, pneumococcus, staphylococcus, diptheria, and hemolytic streptococcus. This oil purifies air and water. Many vitamins are included. This extract lowers blood pressure, is antiseptic, and is able to improve heart function and act as an antidote to poisons.

3. Peppermint — This is known to cause a rapid improvement in mental alertness. This relieves nausea, fever, vomiting, indigestion, heartburn, and kills intestinal parasites as well as many bacteria. It is used for asthma, bronchitis, and sinusitis as well as for relief of pain.

4. Purification — This is a blend of Citronella, Lemongrass, Lavendin, and Melaleuca. This was developed to purify air of pathogens, neutralize mildew, cigarette smoke, and other home and office odors.

5. Joy — This blend has Ylang ylang, Bergamot, Citrus, and Turkish rose oil. This was developed to relax the body and mind. Ylang ylang lowers blood pressure. Bergamot has a long history of use for infections. Turkish rose has the highest electrical frequency of all essential oils (320 Hz.). This is good for infections and stimulates and elevates the mind.

6. Peace and Calming — This blend includes Citrus, Ylang Ylang, Tanactum, and Patchouly. This was developed to calm after a stressful day. When diffused in the home it relaxes overactive and hard to manage children. This is very effective for insomnia.

7. Pan Away — This blend contains Helichrysum, Birch, Clove, and Peppermint. This was developed by Young to reduce inflammation and relieve pain. Clove has been used in European hospitals for viral hepatitis, colitis, cholera, amebiasis, sinusitis, bronchitis, tuberculosis, and thyroid dysfunction.

If you are unfamiliar with essential oils, the Essential 7 kit discusssed above would be a good place to start. This comes with an Essential Oils Symptoms Guide.

We highly recommend Young Living Essential Oils which can be purchased from Sunshine Team 888-322-6271 and *from Natural Health Team* 800-416-2806.

Aroma Therapy For High Blood Pressure

For those of you who dislike taking pills, aroma therapy may be just the answer. This therapy is a blended essential oil derived from the ylang ylang tree. Essential oils are very potent and must not be taken orally.

Dr. Marcial-Vega, a recognized pioneer in this field, has noted an 80% favorable response in patients with hypertension. Two thirds of patients with severe high blood pressure (malignant hypertension) responded favorably.

One drop of the oil is placed on a finger on one hand and the fingers are rubbed together. The aroma is inhaled for one minute. The blood pressure stays down for an average of ten hours.

Obviously, you will need an electronic blood pressure cuff or a conventional blood pressure cuff to determine if a blood pressure fall is occurring and how long it is lasting. The inhalation treatment will need to be repeated when the blood pressure starts to rise. If the blood pressure does not drop, add one more drop to the quantity being rubbed before inhalation. The rubbing warms the oil and improves the effect. Persons taking ylang ylang Essential Oils for hypertension will avoid any drug side effects.

Blended ylang ylang oil can be obtained from Health Horizons 800 771 - 0255 or 305 442- 1233 and from *Natural Health Team* 800-416-2806.

The Grave Danger Of Hydrogenated Fat

In the modern way to make food, an unnatural fat called trans fat or *hydrogenated fat* is created when the unsaturated vegetable oil is given two hydrogen atoms to increase stability and shelf life.

This addition of hydrogen atoms occurs during high temperature conditions and addition of chemicals. The resultant sludge not only has no nutritional value but also *is extremely dangerous because it behaves like a saturated fat in causing arteriosclerotic plaques to form with greatly increased risk of heart disease in persons eating these trans fats. These abnormal fats are found in nearly 100% of packaged foods including cake mixes, crackers, breakfast cereals, microwave pop corn, mayonnaise, salad oils, cooking oils and margarine.*

Butter is far safer than margarine. I encourage you to read the labels on the foods you buy. When you see hydrogenated, partially hydrogenated, and polyunsaturated oils, consider purchasing other products. You will be surprised at how few remain.

When their sales go down, the food manufacturers may give us food that has *real* soybeans, corn, safflower, peanut, canola and sunflower ingredients that will be infinitely safer. *Probably smaller, innovative companies will seize the opportunity to create truly safe foods.*

Exercise

All patients with heart disease do better with exercise; even patients with congestive heart failure who can only do light exertion. Non-exerting heart patients are vulnerable to blood clots in leg veins, which can be fatal.

Regular exercise strengthens the heart, lowers blood pressure, and improves the circulation. The cholesterol and triglycerides fall and the *good* HDL rises.

The risk of heart attack goes down and the person who exercises is more likely to survive a heart attack. Exercise also improves carbohydrate metabolism and wards off the development of type 2 diabetes.

Thirty minutes daily of brisk walking is believed to be adequate. With regular sustained exercise, the heart pumps more blood with each heartbeat, the lungs supply more oxygen to the blood and the arteries deliver more blood to the tissues. The end result is more work accomplished with less effort.

An added benefit of exertion is the release from the brain of mood elevating endorphins. These endorphins start to be released after 20 minutes of exercise and continue their action for hours after the exertion.

An interesting study from Hawaii disclosed that a group of men over the age of 71 who walked one and one half miles daily were 50% less likely to experience a heart attack than elderly males who walked less than one half mile daily.

Violent physical exertion such as marathon running and professional athletics causes the release of enormous amounts of free radicals. When marathon runners are not taking enough antioxidants or are taking the wrong antioxidants, this massive free radical release causes accelerated injury to arteries with extensive arteriosclerosis and may predispose to the development of cancer. Large amounts of vitamin E, magnesium and a readily absorbed form of CoQ10 are the most frequently lacking supplements in these individuals.

Valuable Supplements For Heart Patients

Vitamin C

Free radicals are toxic to cell membranes, proteins, chromosomes, and DNA. Their attack on DNA can lead to mutations that result in cancer.

Uncontrolled, these free radicals damage arterial walls, which then develop cholesterol plaques. Antioxidants like Vitamin C decrease the dangerous action of free radicals on Lipoprotein(a) causing it to stick to an artery wall where the lining is injured. Vitamin C has an important role in moving to these areas of artery damage and works to repair the injury. Vitamin C is 95% effective in blocking cholesterol plaque formation.

Vitamin E

A low level of Vitamin E in the blood was more than twice as reliable in predicting a forthcoming heart attack as was high cholesterol or elevated blood pressure. That's how vital Vitamin E is. 400 mg. daily is needed and 800 mg. is probably even better.

A population study in 1996 was published in *Lancet* (a British medical journal). In this study of 2002 patients with heart disease, half were given 400 mg. or 800 mg. of Vitamin E whereas the other half were given a placebo. After 510 days the results showed 75% fewer heart attacks in the group getting Vitamin E.

An earlier study of 87,245 nurses and 46,000 physicians revealed that those taking as little as 100 units of vitamin E daily had 40% and 37% lower rates of heart attack and death from heart disease than those on no vitamin E.

Beta Carotene

Beta carotene neutralizes singlet oxygen which gets stopped from forming more toxic free radicals. 10,000 to 15000 IU are needed daily. Beta carotene is a precursor to Vitamin A. Vitamin A can be toxic in excessively large amounts (50,000 units daily for one year).

Arteriosclerosis Caused By Hyperhomocysteinemia And Its Correction

Dr. Kilmer McCulley is responsible for the discovering that elevated levels of homocysteine damage arteries. Homocysteine stops the production of the valuable vasodilating nitric acid, causes blood to thicken, and facilitates the oxidation of LDL cholesterol, thus setting the stage for an atherosclerotic plaque to form. *As more patients are studied it has become evident that elevated levels of homocysteine are a common cause for arteriosclerosis (40%).*

If you have artery problems, measuring homocysteine in the blood will frequently provide clear evidence that *homocysteine* is causing the problem, not cholesterol.

A Norwegian study published in the New England Journal of Medicine on July 24,1997 discovered that in 587 patients with coronary heart disease *the risk of death within four years was proportional to total plasma homocysteine level* . The risk rose from 3.8% with homocysteine below 9 micromols per liter to 24.7% in patients with homocysteine levels above 15 micromols per liter.

The only way to be certain that you are getting the proper dosage of folic acid, Vitamin B 12, Vitamin B6 and Trimethylglycine to treat homocysteine excess is to have regular tests of homocysteine (HC) blood levels. Each 3 unit increase in HC causes a 35% increase in the risk of heart attack.

Trimethylglycine (TMG) is the most effective agent to lower homocysteine levels. (Page 86 of Disease Prevention and Treatment: Third Edition). The usual dose is 500 mg. three times daily. If HC levels have not fallen adequately, up to 9000 mg.. of TMG may be needed daily.

Folic acid (800 mcg with each meal) and 1000 mcg. of B 12 daily is also needed.

B6 (pyridoxine) reduces HC by a different method than folic acid. The dose of B6 should be 100 to 200 mg. daily.

In a patient with previous bypass surgery, angina reappeared along with new areas of blockage of heart arteries. This man was taking 15,000mcg. of folic acid daily. His blood HC level was very high risk at 18. On 6 grams daily of trimethylglycine, his HC fell to 4 in one month.

Trimethylglycine functions in treating elevated HC levels by donating methyl groups, which convert HC to the harmless aminoacid methionine.

Trimethylglycine(Betaine) can be purchased in health food stores.

Essential Fatty Acids

Omega 3 and Omega 6 fatty acids have important roles to play in the immune system, inflammation, blood flow, blood clotting, and blood pressure. Research at the University of Oregon found that 10 patients with very high triglyceride levels had their triglyceride levels fall from 1,353mg.% to 281mg.% and the cholesterol fell from 373mg.% to 207 mg. on a diet high in fish oil.

Taking 2 to 10 fish oil capsules and 2 tablespoons of flax oil or ¼ cup of ground flax seed daily is sufficient to improve blood lipids.

Lecithin

Lecithin is a perfect example of a key health component accomplishing much for very little expense. At one time lecithin was the foundation of all treatment programs dealing with circulation problems This substance has great value in both preventing and treating cardiovascular problems.

Lecithin is a combination of phosphatidylcholine (PC) which is 23% of the total weight of lecithin and choline which makes up 13% of the total weight. Lecithin is found in the high cholesterol high fat foods (fatty beef steak, beef liver and eggs) all of which are eaten less than previously.

Lecithin lowers the bad LDL cholesterol and raised the good HDL cholesterol. This occurs by two mechanisms: decreasing cholesterol absorption from the gut and actually pulling harmful forms of cholesterol out of the blood stream. The choline component in lecithin becomes metabolized into betaine, which is able to lower homocysteine blood levels and thus help to prevent arteriosclerosis.

The liver plays a critical role in getting rid of dangerous chemical toxins and pesticides. Abnormal liver function, liver enlargement and fat replacement of liver tissue can be caused by viral and other infections, cancer, alcohol abuse, exposure to chemical toxins and choline deficient diets. Increasing lecithin intake appears to be vital in minimizing liver damage (Gastroenterology 92:102: 1363-70).

The phosphatidylcholine (PC) component of lecithin appears to be responsible for protecting the liver. Usually the liver produces an enzyme that helps the liver make PC. Alcoholics have an inadequate supply of this enzyme and thus fail to produce the proper amount of PC. Use of either PC or lecithin in the diet may prevent alcohol induced cirrhosis and liver damage.

Nerve cells meet at junctions called synapses. In these sites a chemical compound called acetylcholine (AC) is often used to transmit the nerve impulses. These synapses are most frequent in the brain. To produce AC the nerve cells need choline. This can be created from other compounds by the nerve cell, or derived from breakdown of their own cell membranes but the preferable course is to get choline directly from the blood stream. Daily ingestion of lecithin causes the AC levels in the brain to rise. This is very beneficial.

When a group of older persons took two tablespoons of lecithin daily for five weeks they exhibited fewer memory lapses and improve memory skills (Res. Social Work Practice 94:4:349-58). Another study involving college students revealed that taking a high dose of lecithin (10 grams) could significantly improve short term memory skills within 90 minutes of consumption (Clin Neuopharm 93:16 (6): 540-9).

It can take months for the body to build up a reserve of the fat-like components of lecithin. Therefore, if you want to experience the full benefits of lecithin it must be taken regularly for months. Lecithin clearly has positive effects on the memory and numerous other benefits. It has no known side effect.

For daily maintenance purposes one tablespoon (2 grams) of lecithin is adequate. To treat severe heart disease, high cholesterol, abnormal liver function and liver disease requires up to 5 to 20 tablespoons (10 to 40 grams) spread throughout the day. Keep the granules in the refrigerator to prevent the development of rancidity.

Lecithin is available through health food stores or Branson Laboratories 800 235 3200

L-Arginine

Arteriosclerosis begins with an injury to the endothelial cell lining a blood vessel. High blood pressure, cholesterol elevation, or cigarette smoke can initiate this process. This injury permits liporotein (a), cholesterol and platelets to clump at the site of injury.

Healthy endothelial cells produce an endothelial relaxing factor (nitric oxide or "*NO*") that prevents the deposition of white blood cells and platelets. If the lining endothelial cells do not have l-arginine, they fail to make *NO*, which may permit a plaque to form that that might lead to a heart attack.

Diseased arteries produce less *NO* than normal arteries. Because these arteries are making less *NO* there is less protection against further damage to the artery. When arginine is taken it increases the *NO* production by the remaining healthy cells in the damaged artery and protects the artery from new plaque formation.

Among the cardiac effects of *NO* are the following:

- Protects the endothelial cells lining the arteries from adherence of plaque.

- In its role as a potent antioxidant it guards LDL (bad cholesterol) from free radicals.

- Prevents platelets from clumping together and thus decreases the formation of clots which helps stop the progressive artery injury problem.

- *NO* is a powerful dilator of blood vessels. When the muscle cells receive instruction from *NO* to relax, the size of the vessel is expanded. Blood can then flow through with less resistance and less pressure exerted against the wall of the artery. This leads to lower blood pressure.

- Two grams of arginine daily can often lower the blood pressure by 20 points in one week.

- When the synthesis of *NO* is blocked, *there is a sharp rise in blood pressure.*

- *NO relaxes arteries and prevents spasm of cardiac arteries which can lead to severe chest pain.*

An important study in the journal *CIRCULATION* showed that *arginine supplementation over time was followed by decrease in size of the arteriosclerotic plaque.*

Because of the beneficial effects on arterial plaques, lowering of blood pressure in hypertensive patients, increasing the output of nitrous oxide which protects arteries from plaque formation, increase in the output of growth hormone and help for many males with impotence, we encourage the use of arginine. Arginine can be obtained from Jo Mar Laboratories 800-538-4545 and from our *Natural Health Team* 800-416-2806..

A dose of arginine of 6 grams taken at bedtime allows *NO* to be restored to artery walls.

Dihydroepiandosterone (DHEA)

DHEA has been studied by Dr. Elizabeth Barrett-Connor at the University of San Diego. DHEA typically falls steadily after the age of 20 to levels in the 70's of only 20% of a 20 year old.

Elevation of the DHEA by 100 mg% in patients with heart disease was associated with a fall in mortality from all causes and a 48% reduction in deaths from cardiovascular disease.

She felt that the reason for this remarkable fact might be that DHEA inhibits the enzyme glucose 6 phosphate dehydrogenase, which is responsible for increasing the production of fatty acids and cholesterol. Keeping the DHEA higher would thus cause less obesity and arteriosclerosis (lower cholesterol).

The usual dose is 50mg. daily in males and 25 mg. daily in females. The correct dosage can only be established by blood tests or saliva tests of DHEA.

DHEA can be obtained in health food stores and from *Natural Health Team* 1-800-4162806.

Chelation

Many of the leaders in the natural health field have great confidence in chelation. In this therapy EDTA (calcium disodium versenate) is slowly infused into the body. The EDTA attaches to minerals (lead, mercury and cadmium) and causes them to be excreted by the kidney.

Recent studies have shown that this form of therapy appears to act as a powerful anti-oxidant. More than 500,000 patients have received this treatment worldwide. Among the conditions that have benefited from this therapy are heart pain (angina pectoris), impaired circulation to the legs, high cholesterol and mental confusion with arteriosclerosis of the arteries to the brain. Possibly when EDTA binds to the calcium deposited in arteries, it removes the deposited calcium and opens up the plaque to being scavenged away. Certainly the anti-oxidant effect of this therapy should permit slow improvement in the arterial circulation.

The therapy involves 20 to 30 intravenous infusions of EDTA with minerals over a period of three to five months. Each infusion should last three to four hours. Kidney function and urine tests need to be followed. Obviously, better results will be found in those who change their lifestyles (stop smoking, control blood pressure, change diet, control cholesterol and homocysteine, exercise etc.) These infusions cost $50 to $100 each, which often is not covered by insurance. When you consider that coronary bypass surgery, stent placement and balloon angioplasty are also expensive, have risks and may need to be repeated, the expense is very reasonable. No deaths have been reported from this therapy.

EECP

This interesting procedure was developed at Harvard Medical School by Dr. Harry Soroff, 43 years ago. The term EECP stands for enhanced external counterpulsion. During the procedure a body stocking, which extends from the ankles to the waist contracts with each heart beat forcing more blood than usual to go to the heart muscle, brain, and body. During the course of 35 one hour treatments given twice daily, there is enough pressure generated against artery walls to open up new blood channels to heart muscle. This therapy was able to eliminate angina in 16 of 18 patients reported in the *American Journal of Cardiology* in 1992.The other two patients were improved, but were not completely free of chest pain.

If you have been told you need angioplasty, which is a procedure in which a blocked artery is forcibly opened by a balloon, stent placement or bypass surgery consider EECP. Angioplasty frequently needs to be repeated and there are significant risks from bypass surgery (emboli to brain, stroke, infarction of heart, decreased mental faculties which is not always temporary, death, and greater expense). Remember, physicians fall into the habit of doing procedures that they are familiar with.

Coronary artery *repair* by angioplasty, stent placement, and coronary artery bypass are procedures that have become a huge industry in the United States. *Unfortunately, in large population studies there is no clear evidence that any of these procedures is any better than good medical management of the patient (proper diet, treatments to correct homocysteine and cholesterol, blood pressure, cigarettes, antioxidants and omega 3 fatty acids.)*

There is one important exception to the remarks about considering medical therapy *instead* of angioplasty, stents or bypass and that is significant left main coronary artery obstruction. *Because most of the blood flow to the heart comes from the left coronary artery, serious obstruction of this artery can cause sudden death.*

Most experts recommend proceeding to coronary artery bypass surgery when left main coronary occlusion is nearly complete.

Angina Pectoris

Angina Pectoris is a very common cardiac condition with 6.5 million people in the USA suffering from it. Patients with angina will experience chest pain after exertion or meals because the heart muscle is not receiving an adequate amount of blood through narrowed cardiac arteries. (Arterioclerosis) With rest, the pain resolves in a few minutes. Standard therapy involves nitroglycerine which gives temporary dilation of the cardiac arteries which relieves the pain.

In a double-blind stury of 50 patients, half received Padma and half a placebo. After two weeks, 80% of the patients getting Padma had experienced good to excellent results. In this short time, the average number of angina attacks was reduced from 37.5 to 11.5. (Source: Herba Polinica 86:32:107-114)

Artery Cleanser (Grapefruit Pectin)

Grapefruit pectin has the ability to prevent arteriosclerosis in pigs, which were made hypercholesterolemic by a special diet. This has potential benefit for humans and is discussed further in Chapter 23 (Arteriosclerosis)

Chapter 5

Diabetes Mellitus

There are two types of diabetes : Type 1 insulin dependent and Type 2 insulin resistant. The patients in Type 1 must take insulin to stay alive, whereas the patients with Type 2 diabetes have high levels of insulin in their blood but are unable to properly utilize insulin to burn sugar.

Diabetes has at least three recognized causes:

Genetic

There is a strong familial tendency to inherit diabetes in some families.

Autoimmune

Many persons have a form of diabetes in which the body develops antibodies against tissues such as the islet cells of the pancreas. As the islet cells are destroyed diabetes appears.

Immunization with vaccines can be promptly followed by the onset of Type 1 diabetes in children. Approximately 80% of children with Type 1 diabetes are believed to have developed the illness from an adverse reaction to a vaccine. The mechanism is believed to be an autoimmune injury to the pancreatic islet cells precipitated by a vaccine. If my child developed Type 1 diabetes from a vaccine, I would give the child a trial of two to three months of thymic extract.

Thymic extract has been shown to be very effective in treating autoimmune disorders. (see Chapter 3 Immune Illnesses) .

Viral Illness

Some persons become diabetic immediately after a viral illness, which has probably seriously injured the pancreas.

In the United States there is an *epidemic* of Type 2 diabetes with estimates of 10% of persons having this illness. An estimated *16 million Americans have Type 2 Diabetes. It strikes 800,000 new victims each year.*

What Is The Cause Of Type 2 Diabetes And How Can It Be Cured?

A 65-year-old electronic engineer named Thomas Smith was discovered to have diabetes with fasting sugars of 350 mg. and sugars after a meal of 550 mg.

He went to a physician and when he learned that there was no cure, he embarked on an extensive literature search to find a cure. After 107 days of learning what to do about diabetes, his blood sugars were back to normal. No drugs or other therapy had been used. He has written a book titled *Insulin: Our Silent Killer* (Phone 866-320 7700 to order) in which he outlines the cause and path to recovery from Type 2 diabetes.

Diabetes was a very rare illness in the United States in 1880, with only 2.8 persons out of every 100,000 having diabetes. Now at least 10% of the populace has diabetes and when you look for early signs of diabetes (hyperinsulinemia) that number is certain to be much higher. What Mr. Smith discovered was that high blood insulin levels preceded the elevation of blood sugar values, on which the diagnosis of diabetes is established.

No one knows how long these blood insulin values are elevated *before* the pancreas fails and the blood sugars begin to rise. What appears to be occurring is that the blood sugar values are maintained at normal values by virtue of excretion of greater and greater quantities of insulin, *until the pancreas fails*. This may well vary considerably in duration from person to person, but the occurrence of *elevated insulin values is the diagnostic clue to the future appearance of diabetes.*

High insulin values decrease the production of HDL (good cholesterol) by inhibiting the enzyme lipoprotein lipase. This leads to lower HDL and a rise in triglycerides and LDL (bad cholesterol).

Rising blood cholesterol and triglycerides may thus be an indicator of insulin excess and might be a clue to future trouble with diabetes. Persons with elevated cholesterol and triglycerides should have their insulin levels checked. High triglyceride values are very common in diabetes. We are accustomed to blaming cholesterol and triglceride problems on heredity, when many really seem to be a consequence of eating the wrong food(no Omega 3 fatty acid and eating dangerous artificial fats).

When the pre diabetic person is experiencing chronic high insulin values, this insulin is converting some of the glucose into the fat triglyceride, which gets stored in fat cells which end up distended in an obese patient.

In this manner, high insulin levels are producing most of our obese persons. Obese persons also need to have insulin levels checked, as many of them are certainly pre diabetic. In England, a long term follow up study in an obesity clinic revealed that all patients eventually became diabetic. A third undesirable effect of high insulin values is the development of lesions in arterial walls called plaques that may lead to strokes, heart attacks, and gangrene.

Features common to Type 2 diabetics are:

- Sedentary Life Style

- High hydrogenated fat intake

- High refined Carbohydrate intake

- Absence of Omega 3 fatty acids in the diet

In Chapter 1, the widespread lack of Omega 3 fatty acids in the American diet was documented.

In the United States there has been a steady shift in type of fat eaten from butter and lard to margarine and chemically manufactured shortenings (Crisco and Snowdrift) and artificial salad oils. This shift accelerated during World War 1 and there was a critical deterioration in health when Archer Daniel Midlands stopped making flax oil in 1950.

At the same time, the U.S. public was being seduced by clever ads depicting saturated fat as bad and the new artificial fats as healthy. *The new fats are transfats, not the polyunsaturated fats of animal and plant origin that are vital to good health.* The high temperatures needed to extract and refine these artificial products destroy all contents of the original food and create synthetic polyunsaturated and monounsatuated fats of artificial origin.

These transfats are very difficult for the body to dispose of in small quantities and certainly cause far greater damage when they are present in large quantities on a daily basis. It is a tribute to the body's amazing healing attributes that we live as long as we do when we are eating so much worthless, synthetic substances.

Meanwhile, major changes were occurring on the nation's farms. The fertilizers used for replenishing the soil contained Nitrogen, Phosphorus, and Potassium. Alfalfa will not grow unless Boron is present in the soil, *so this is supplied. However, the overwhelming majority of farmers never replace trace minerals.*

As long ago as 1936, a U.S. Senate document #264 stated:

"Do most of you know that most of us today are suffering from certain dangerous diet deficiencies which can not be remedied until the depleted soils from which our foods come are brought into a proper mineral balance? The alarming fact is that the foods, fruits, vegetables and grains, now being raised on millions of acres of land that no longer contains enough of certain needed minerals, *are starving us, no matter how much we eat." And that was in 1936! Without the critical trace minerals in our food, carbohydrate metabolism fails.*

Dr. Albrecht, Chairman of the Department of Soils at the University of Missouri, and a legend in his time, once said: "A declining soil fertility, due to lack of organic material, major elements, and trace minerals is responsible for poor crops and in turn for the pathological conditions in animals fed deficient foods from such soils, and that mankind is no exception."

Dr. Albrecht further charged "NPK (nitrogen phosphorous potassium) fertilizer formulas as legislated and enforced by State Department of Agriculture mean malnutrition, attack by insects, bacteria, and fungi, weed takeover of crop loss in dry weather, and *general loss of mental acuity in the population, leading to degenerative metabolic disease and early death."*

Farmers are paid to produce maximum yield per acre of salable produce; they have no incentive to produce nutrition. In the future, farmers will again do well financially when they produce organic foods from soil that contains minerals. More and more consumers will demand healthy food as they realize their lives are in jeopardy from the chemically dependent agribusiness products.

In 1992, the earth summit report reviewed the extent to which the world's farmland had been depleted. Of all continents, North America was the most seriously depleted. *Our soil has lost 85% of its mineral content through the modern farm practices.* Most continents were in the mid 70th percentile.

Back in 1963, Dr. Jerome Weisner, Science Counselor to President Kennedy, stated *"the farm use of pesticides is more dangerous than atomic fallout"*.

Of great import to the diabetic is the following information:

Processed food contains pesticide residues and additives.

 Processed food is *loaded* with artificial fat, sugar, artificial sweeteners, and other artificial ingredients.

The food processing industry makes wide use of subliminal technology in promoting their products.

The large quantity of synthetic fats and oil, as well as sugar that are added to processed food, are particularly damaging to the diabetic's ability to control his blood sugar.

Cellular membrane dysfunction occurs when the body must manufacture and repair our cell membranes with the wrong fatty acids, because the right ones are not available from our diet. Our cellular membranes require Omega 3 fatty acids for proper functioning.

There is no doubt that the refined oils, hydrogenated fats, and a severe lack of the Omega 3 fatty acids are contributing to our diabetes epidemic. The control of blood sugar depends on adequate amounts of the minerals zinc, chromium, vanadium, and magnesium, which are lacking in the foods grown in soil treated with Phosphorus, Nitrogen, and Potassium fertilizer used by most farmers. We are being poisoned by pesticides, lack of essential fatty acids, toxic trans fat isomers and toxic additives. Diabetics have the additional problem that they are losing large quantities of minerals and vitamins in their urine whenever their blood sugars are elevated.

Is there any wonder there is an epidemic of Type 2 Diabetes, with 16 million victims and 800,000 being added each year?

How Can The Diabetic Recover From Type 2 Diabetes?

There are three key components needed for recovery from Type 2 diabetes:

Begin Omega 3 fatty acid therapy daily

Start with either 2 tablespoons of flax oil or 4 tablespoons of ground flax seed daily. Omega 3 fatty acids play a critical role in healing the damaged cell membranes which have interfered with the movement of glucose into the cell.

Eliminate all synthetic (manufactured) fat from your diet.

This includes all processed foods found in boxes, packages, cans and wrappers. Study these and you will discover they all contain hydrogenated, partially hydrogenated or polyunsaturated artificial fats. Often they may be labeled as polyunsaturated or monounsaturated soy, corn, saffola, canola, peanut or sunfloweroil. These substances are manufactured in a factory at high temperatures and contain dangerous trans fats that are difficult for the immune system to eliminate from the body. They cause elevation of low density (bad) cholesterol leading to arteriosclerosis.

Restrict your fat intake to between 15 to 25% of your total calories.

One of the characteristics of the Type 2 diabetic is failure to progress into severe ketoacidosis, which is a medical emergency. This has been attributed to the presence of small amounts of residual insulin sufficient to prevent ketosis. *This residual insulin is adequate to control blood sugar if the fat intake in restricted.* As soon as the dietary fat intake is violated there will be prompt reappearance of elevated blood sugar values and the dangerous hyperinsulinemia with the risk of arterial narrowing. *Remember high insulin levels are just as dangerous as high blood sugar levels.*

Initially all sugar needs to be eliminated. This impedes the liver's ability to transform sugar into fat. Remember, when blood sugar levels are returned to normal the insulin blood level is often still elevated. High blood insulin levels are implicated in damage to arteries. Later when glucose control is well established you can add brown sugar for flavoring, dates, stevia and honey in small quantities. When sugar is added prematurely the blood sugars rise and the recovery is set back in time. Obese patients take longer to recover blood sugar control possibly because they have larger fat reserves than thin persons. These large fat reserves contain abnormal trans fats, which may still be used in building cell membranes. When these abnormal fats have been totally metabolized away the membranes will be normal.

Another condition afflicting the Type 2 diabetic is non ketotic hyperosmolar coma. In this condition high blood sugar values cause the steady daily loss of sugar and large amounts of fluid in the urine. This eventually results in such severe fluid lack that brain function becomes impaired with confusion, stupor and progression to coma. Hospital therapy consists of restoring the huge fluid and electrolytes deficit along with insulin.

To be successful in ridding yourself of Type 2 diabetes you must change what you eat. If you continue to believe that "I deserve a break today" you will have great difficulty curing this disease.

You must immediately stop eating all processed food. You will need to become an expert at reading labels, looking for sugar, hydrogenated fat, partially hydrogenated fat, polyunsaturated fat, refined fat, preservatives and colorants. This means that nearly all food found in cans, boxes, packages and bottles are going to be perpetuating the diabetic state if consumed. *The exclusion of synthetic fats from your diet needs to be permanent.*

An intelligent dietician who understands the danger of synthetic fats can be a valuable asset. Assistance in planning meals so that total fat intake daily does not exceed 25% will be of great value. The last one half of Dr. Julian Whitaker's book *Reversing Diabetes* contains a detailed 30 day menu guideline for the preparation of delicious meals that are low in fat.

Take 2 to 3 tablespoons of flax oil or 4 tablespoons of ground flax seed daily. This must be cold pressed. This means the oil was removed at temperatures less than 110 degree Fahrenheit.

Keep fat intake severely restricted until the blood sugar has returned to normal *(fasting blood sugar below 100mg. seven days in a row.)* During this period the body cell membranes are being repaired. At that point, slowly add back small quantities of butter, coconut oil, virgin olive oil and clean lard.

To maintain normal blood sugar values, the dietary fat intake needs to be maintained in the 15 to 25% range, far less than the average American's 45% level.

Supplements are very important, including the minerals chromium picolate 300 mg. three times daily, vanadium 100mcg. daily, copper 3 mg. daily, calcium 1000 mg. daily, magnesium 500 mg. daily, manganese 30 mg. daily, molybedenum 200 mcg. daily, manganese 30 mg daily, selenium 200 mcg. daily, zinc 50 mg. three times daily, iodine 150 mcm. daily, sulfur 500 mg. daily, boron 3 to 9 mg. daily, and silicon 10 mg. daily.

Vitamins that are needed include Vitamin A 5000 IU, Vitamin D 400 IU, B1 (thiamine) 100 mg., B2 riboflavin 10 mg., B3 niacinamide 50 mg. three times daily, Inositol Hexaniacianate 400 mg. three times daily, B 5 pantothene 300mg. three times daily, B6 pyridoxine 100 mg daily, B 12 2000 mcg. daily, Vitamin C 600 mg. three times daily, carotenes 25,000 IU, mixed E tocopherols 400 IU three times daily, biotin 10 mg. daily, phosphatidylcholine 500 mg. three times daily, folic acid 400 mg. daily and bioflavinoids from bilberry or grape seed 500 mg. three times daily.

Other nutrients of value include alpha lipoic acid 600 mg. daily, Quercetin 200 mg. three times daily, CoQ10 120 mg. daily, l-carnitine 100 mg. daily.

Exercise will be of great value in assisting blood sugar return. Spend 15 to 20 minutes daily three times daily ideally after meals unless you have angina from eating food.

Develop new dietary habits:

No frozen convenience foods. No deep-fried foods. No fatty foods, No fortified foods. No fast foods. No fake foods. No artificial flavors. No machine fabricated foods.

Less than 10% of the aisles in the grocery will contain something suitable. You will be shocked to learn that nearly all supermarket food has added sugar and synthetic fats. Nearly everything in a can, box, bottle or package has artificial fat and sugar. (Mr. Smith buys a side a beef from a farmer who raises cattle without hormones and stores this in his freezer.) Patronize health food stores and organic food stores. Try to eat cold food, which has all it's nutrients intact. Bake and broil, avoiding frying if at all possible.

If you have a tiny bit of land, grow your own organic produce (see chapter 35 for an exciting way to greatly increase yield of more nutritious food). Patronize farmers who give you nutritious organic food. If you follow this program, you have an opportunity to *permanently* recover from your Type 2 diabetes. Unfortunately, there will be some individuals who value their artificial food more than returning to good health. Others may find the effort to find safe food too bothersome.

The fact that cholesterol elevation can be corrected in many patients with flax oil suggests that much of the problem with cholesterol is due to lack of Omega 3 fatty acids and a glut of artificial fat in the diet *and is not genetic.* We strongly urge those of you with type 2 diabetes to start flax oil or perilla oil. Get rid of the artificial fats in your diet, as uncorrected diabetes is a killer with a greatly shortened life expectancy.

Because of this information about insulin, we think including an insulin blood level in the annual examination is very desirable. *The detection of hyperinsulinemia from this test gives an earlier warning than previously available that diabetes is ahead, unless drastic life style changes are made.*

Thomas Smith is no longer a diabetic as long as he stays away from the harmful fats that caused his illness, continues to supply his body with Omega 3 fatty acid (flax oil, fish oil or perilla oil), and restricts total daily fat intake to less than 25% of total calories. When he has dietary indiscretions and his fasting blood sugar starts to rise towards 100mg., he immediately returns to very serious restriction of synthetic and total fat.

To summarize: Type 2 diabetes appears to be an illness caused by abnormal fat metabolism induced by absence of Omega 3 fatty acids and the presence of dangerous artificial fats in the diet. *Omega 3 fatty acids are responsible for the maintenance and repair of cellular membranes. When the body lacks Omega 3 fatty acids the omega 6 and omega 9 fatty acids must be used.* This results in a stiff and sticky cell membrane, instead of the usual slippery and smooth membrane. These abnormal membranes do not permit easy transport of glucose into the cell and the blood sugar stays high.

The disease is reversible with appropriate dietary changes in approximately 90% of cases.

In the early stage of this illness, high levels of insulin are a warning that eventually high blood sugars will appear. Elevated cholesterol and triglyceride values, obesity, hypertension, and the clinical appearance of vascular damage are all clues that point toward a pre-diabetic state. This diagnosis can be confirmed by the finding of high insulin levels in the blood. *When a population study of insulin levels is done in hypertensive, obese, hypercholestertolemic, hypertriglyceridemic, and arteriosclerotic patients we may discover that up to 20% of the U.S populace are pre diabetic.*

We owe a debt of gratitude to Thomas Smith for his relentless pursuit of the cause of his Type 2 diabetes. He's not a doctor. He is an intelligent engineer who used an intensive literature search to learn how to correct his diabetes.

Exertion

A critical cornerstone in the management of diabetes is regular exertion. Obtaining an exercise treadmill test prior to beginning an exercise program is *very* important. That's because diabetics are notorious for having a high degree of damage to heart arteries *without any warning symptoms. Unfortunately, the proof of having serious narrowing may be sudden death after vigorous exertion.* This artery narrowing can usually be detected by the abnormalities seen in the electrocardiogram during the exercise treadmill test.

Moderate exercise has a more intense effect in lowering blood sugar levels in diabetics than it does in normal persons. Eight to ten minutes of exertion immediately after meals tends to keep the blood sugar at lower levels all day long. This should be avoided for two or three hours, if eating is known to bring on chest pain (angina).

The long-term benefit of regular exercise is to increase the body's sensitivity to the insulin still being produced by the body or the insulin injected as part of the treatment program.

One benefit of exercise is a decrease in the abnormal increased stickiness of platelets often seen in diabetics. This increased stickiness of platelets contributes to the excessive blood clots so common in diabetic arteries. When your blood has become less sticky, you are less likely to have a heart attack or stroke.

Exercise releases endorphins in the brain and we feel better for several hours.

Exercise is one of the few things that invariably elevates the HDL by a few milligrams. Each 1 mg elevation in HDL level accomplished, *decreases* the chance of a heart attack by 2%. There is a limit to the elevation of HDL that appears after exertion, but even a three or four mg. rise tips the scale of good health toward the individual who exercises. In addition, triglyceride levels fall by substantial amounts after regular exercise.

The heart is greatly helped by regular exercise:

The resting heart rate falls.

A well-conditioned heart accomplishes greater heart rates after exertion than a non-conditioned heart. Thus when more blood is needed, it is properly delivered by the well-conditioned heart.

The well-conditioned heart pumps a greater volume of blood with each heartbeat. This means that exercise training enables greater volumes of blood to be delivered than can be accomplished by the unconditioned heart.

The heart muscle improves it's ability to extract oxygen after exercise training, which is very important to the diabetic because the diabetic often has narrowed arteries to heart muscle.

An important study was performed by Dr. Lyle Peterson, Director of the Comprehensive Rehabilitation Center in Houston, Texas. In this study 12 individuals waiting for heart transplantation were placed in a mild exercise program. These persons were very ill and required close monitoring during all exertion. *To everyone's amazement, 6 of the 12 improved so much they were removed from the heart transplant program and went home to lead essentially normal lives.*

One of the vital accomplishments resulting from regular exertion is the slow steady development of new small blood vessels in the area of major artery narrowing (collateral circulation).

This is often so successful that complete occlusion of the large artery does not cause a heart attack. Exercise is the only activity that leads to the development of collateral blood vessels.

The type of exercise could be walking, bicycling, swimming, or slow jogging. Mild weight lifting can increase total muscle mass and be beneficial in cutting insulin resistance. Having a larger muscle mass permits disposal of more sugar during exertion. Walking is safe and inexpensive. Try to go 1 ½- 2 miles daily, 6 days a week.

An exertion study was done in sixteen out of shape men who had insulin resistance and were at risk for diabetes. Eight men were given aerobic exercise and eight men were given the same aerobic exercise followed by one hour of strength training (weight lifting). There were reductions in insulin levels, decrease in blood sugar and lower blood pressure in all 16 men.

However, the men receiving the strength training lowered their insulin levels three times as much as the aerobics only group and their glucose and blood pressure decreased by twice as much.

There is a dangerous tendency on the part of diabetic patients that needs to be addressed. Often the diabetic wants a "magic bullet pill", so he can eat the same way he wants to and remain indolent, depending on the magic drug bullet to correct the diabetic problem. *This will not happen.*

Oral Diabetic Pills

When pills to control blood sugar elevations became available they were eagerly accepted, as no diabetics wanted to receive daily injections of insulin. They hoped the pills might lower blood sugar values to acceptable levels where dietary restrictions could be ignored.

Most of these drugs are from the sulfonylurea chemical family including Orinase (tolbutamide), Diabenese (chlorpropamide), Diabeta and Glucatrol (glyburide), and Micronase (glipizide). In 1961, 1027 patients were enrolled in a large study (University Group Diabetes Program) to evaluate whether control of blood sugar with pills or insulin in Type 2 diabetics reduced the frequency of heart disease. Some patients were given Orinase and others received an identical placebo pill. This study was terminated in 8 years because the death rate from heart disease in the patients on oral sulfonylurea (Orinase) was too high.

There were 250% more deaths in the patients receiving Orinase than those getting a placebo. This translates into a one per cent increase in deaths every year among those being treated with Orinase. If 10 million persons have diabetes treated in this manner, this would lead to 100,000 added deaths each year or one million deaths over a 10 year period.

Because physicians were unwilling to accept this data, (because sulphonylureas were the only readily available oral treatment short of insulin that corrected the blood sugar) the use of oral agents continued.

Study of this type of therapy disclosed that the sulfonylureas appear to increase the oxygen demand in the heart thus causing extra work for the heart. Since many diabetics already had a compromised blood flow to the heart muscle by virtue of their arteriosclerosis, this *extra* cardiac work load proved to be a grave problem. There was also a tendency toward irregular heart rhythms, which is dangerous in persons with heart disease. A third potential risk was an apparent lowering of HDL (good cholesterol), which would tend to accelerate artery damage. This evidence about adverse survival in persons on sulfonylureas should bring ready acceptance to any safe new treatments.

Obviously, recovery from Type 2 diabetes should be the goal of every Type 2 diabetic. This may well be possible using Omega 3 fatty acids (flax and perilla oils), avoiding all artificial fats and restricting fat intake to below 25% of total calories daily. It appears that 90% of diabetics who make a serious effort to change their dietary fat problem will succeed in restoring glucose values to normal.

For those who are unwilling to give up faulty dietary habits or who do not achieve a total disappearance of Type 2 diabetes with the proper dietary fat changes, there are some valuable approaches to therapy now available that should enable many diabetics to discontinue sulfonylurea type drugs and metformin. Getting rid of these categories of drugs should improve survival rates.

Many exciting new products are available to treat diabetes. One is:

Alpha Lipoic Acid

Alpha Lipoic Acid (ALA) is a powerful antioxidant. Alpha lipoic acid can get rid of both *fat and water soluble free radicals, which is unique among antioxidants*. ALA has the capability of prolonging and increasing the action of both Vitamin E and Vitamin C. Additionally, ALA by elevating glutathione recycles Vitamin E. Low levels of glutathione, are believed to permit more oxidative damage to cells resulting in neuropathy, inflammation, and damage to organs.

ALA has been used in Germany to treat diabetes for 30 years. There are 4 valuable properties of ALA in diabetic treatment:

• Increases the ability of insulin to burn up glucose.

• ALA decreases insulin resistance. Insulin resistance is an important problem in diabetes. When a patient develops insulin resistance, insulin does not work so glucose does not enter the cell where it should be metabolized, with a fall in glucose levels. Instead, the blood levels of insulin remain high, but the blood sugar does not fall. This is very common in obese diabetics.

• ALA increases ATP production.

- ALA reverses the damage to nerves and eyes in some patients when used in high doses. *This is extremely important, because the diabetic patient develops damage to small blood vessels in the eye, kidney, and nerves (Microangiopathy).* As this microangiopathy progresses, there is loss of sight, painful burning and numbness in the legs, usually worse at night, and gradual decrease in kidney function. This eventually results in uremia, requiring dialysis or transplantation, if it does not cause death.

Dr. D. Zeigler, at the Heinrich-Heine University in Dusseldorf, reported that long term treatment with high dosage ALA induced regeneration of nerves (sprouting). Some patients began to experience decrease in pain and numbness as soon as three weeks after the onset of high dosage ALA treatment. The regeneration has been attributed to improvement in nerve membrane fluidity.

This response in neuropathy and retinitis is very encouraging, as the diabetic problem can apparently be reversed. We suggest the following:

All diabetics with microangiopathy should be treated with 600 to 800 mg. of ALA daily. Doses as high as 1800mg. have been used. Diabetics should get regular checks for urinary microalbumin, as this is an early indicator of kidney damage from diabetes. Annual eye exams are a must to detect early retinal damage.

Anyone who has had diabetes for more than a few years, even with no clinical evidence of kidney, eye or nerve damage *might be prevented from getting diabetic complications by getting started on 100 mg of ALA daily. The complications of diabetes are so devastating (blindness, severe pain and loss of feeling in extremities, and uremia leading to dialysis) that prevention of complications is well worth the effort.*

All other nerve diseases of unknown cause, and alcoholic neuritis, could receive several months of ALA, probably in high dosage, to see if improvement occurs.

Other neurologic diseases of unknown etiology might be tried with 2 months of ALA, as some of them could have a metabolic cause which might be helped by ALA (Guillan Barre,) etc.

It is imperative that diabetic patients receiving ALA be observed by a physician in order to monitor their diabetes, as insulin and or oral diabetic dosage may need to be decreased.

There are no known harmful side effects to ALA. ALA is available at your health food store or from our *Natural Health Team* 800-416-2806.

Gymnema Sylvestre (GS)

Animal experiments have shown that animals which have their Beta cells destroyed by alloxan are able to regenerate Beta cells after a few months when taking GS, a herb grown in India. The Beta cell is the cell that produces insulin. Diabetics needing insulin treatment (Type 1) have been able to decrease their insulin after GS therapy.

Antibetic: This compound contains 10 herbs including GS, all of which have been tested and found to exhibit a lowering of the blood sugar. *Antibetic* has brought about a fall in blood sugar in many patients. Some insulin using diabetics have been able to cut their insulin dosage and a few have been able to stop insulin.

Patients taking diabetic pills have also responded favorably. Obviously patients on this agent will need to have their diabetic treatment monitored by a physician. No serious side effects have been noted.

Antibetic can be obtained from Gero Vital Laboratories at 800-524-9896.

High Complex Carbohydrate Diet

Dr. James Anderson at the University of Kentucky Medical School popularized the high complex carbohydrate, high fiber diet for the treatment of diabetes. With this diet, about 70% of diabetic patients were able to stop insulin and oral diabetic therapy. *This program of bread, pasta, fruit, and vegetables works because fat interferes with the action of insulin while high carbohydrate foods intensify the action of insulin.* Beans seem to be particularly effective in this diet. The carbohydrates used must be natural. Whole-wheat flour is good; white flour is bad.

Valuable Nutrients for Diabetics

People with poorly controlled diabetes are injured by the loss of nutrients in large volumes of urine. The large urine volumes are caused by high blood sugars, which results in glucose spilling into the urine. The presence of large amounts of glucose in the urine has an osmotic effect. In this situation glucose "clings" to magnesium, potassium, and sodium causing them to be lost in the urine along with sugar and vitamins, instead of being normally reabsorbed by the kidney tubules. This means that poorly controlled diabetics waste important products (trace minerals, sugar, sodium, potassium and magnesium) *and need extra supplements to stay in proper metabolic balance.*

Vitamins B 1,B 6, B 12, along with the minerals Vanadium, Magnesium, Zinc, and Chromium are likely to be lacking. Some of the damage to nerves, eyes, arteries and kidneys, could be related to these deficiencies. Important antioxidants such as Vitamin C and E, beta-carotene, and B complex are *essential* for normal carbohydrate and fat metabolism. *Be sure you are on a good vitamin program.*

Ninety per cent of diabetics are deficient in magnesium. Chromium also needs extra supplements. Chromium increases the sensitivity to insulin, which helps lower glucose levels.

Vanadium is a valuable agent for diabetics, as it decreases their need for insulin. Large doses of Vanadium act like an oral insulin. Begin with 45 mg. daily and work the dose up to 100 to 150 mg. daily. A physician's help will be needed to monitor this. Gastrointestinal symptoms may require dose decrease or temporary cessation.

Banaba Therapy

An extract of the leaves of the banaba plant has a material called corosolic acid that lowers blood sugar values in diabetics. When taken in a dose of 48 mg daily 20 diabetics were reported by William Judy, Ph.D to exhibit decrease in sugar levels by 32%. This plant appears to work by increasing the rate that glucose is transported out of the blood. There was no evidence of hypoglycemia.

Glucosol (banaba) can be obtained from Harmony Co. 800-422 5518

Glucose Essentials

Glucose Essentials contains chromium polynicotinate 67 mg., gymnema sylvestre extract 133 mg., banaba leaf extract 5 mg., Siberian ginseng extract 67 mg., holy basil extract 67 mg., vanadyl sulfate 33 mg., green tea 33 mg., bitter melon extract 67mg., and cinnamon bark 100 mg.

All components in the capsule have beneficial effects on glucose metabolism. The dose is three pills daily. This can be obtained from Healthy Directions Inc. 800- 722-8008.

Chapter 6

Rheumatoid Arthritis And Osteoarthritis

Rheumatoid arthritis is an acute inflammatory arthritis characterized by swelling, warmth, and redness of the involved joints. The disease is more common in women than men.

Flare- ups of the illness often occur in winter (cold) months. Studies of 143 women with this condition revealed that Vitamin D levels were subnormal in most persons. Most dietary vitamin D intake in the USA comes from fortified dairy products, margarine, eggs, fish and fish oil. Currently consumption of all these foods, with the exception of fish, is decreasing.

This leaves *sunlight* as the last remaining source for vitamin D. Rheumatoid arthritic patients are likely to be helped by winter exposure to one half hour of sunlight three or four times weekly, without sunscreens.

In addition to getting exposure to sunlight, patients with rheumatoid arthritis *will benefit from changing their food intake to a near vegetarian diet with much less animal protein.*

The other common arthritic problem is osteoarthritis. This appears in everyone just from the simple using of our joints for many years, causing fraying of the cartilage followed by some bony overgrowth. This will be more severe in joints that have been overused and in joints that were injured in the past. There is also a genetic component, as some families are plagued with severe osteoarthritis (OA).

Severely damaged arthritic joints from either rheumatoid arthritis or osteoarthritis may need surgical replacement if they are very painful.

Natural Solutions

THYMIC EXTRACT: (See Chapter 3 for information about thymic extract, which has brought 28 cases of rheumatoid arthritis into an arrested state.)

LYPRINOL: The Maori indigenous populace of New Zealand were recognized to have a very low incidence of arthritic disorders. They attributed their absence of arthritic problems to a large intake of green lipped mussels (lyprinol) from the coast.

After several improvements, this mussel extract was tested against salmon oil, MaxEPA, evening primrose oil and flax oil. It was found to be 150 times more potent than MaxEPA, 240 times more potent than Norwegian salmon oil, 300 times more potent than evening primrose oil and 3,900 times more potent than flax oil in treating inflammation of joints.

Lyprinol was then found to be slightly more effective in treating inflammation than indomethecin or ibuprofen.

Further research has revealed that lyprinol inhibits the 5 lipooxygenase pathway of prostaglandins. All other anti -inflammatory agents block the cyclo-oxygenase pathway.

Lyprinol was the therapy that enabled 5 of my severe rheumatoid arthritis patients to discontinue methotrexate treatment.

This can be obtained from Life Plus 800-572 8446

GLUCOSAMINE AND CHONDROTIN SULPHATE: Both these agents have a clearly established benefit in treating both Rheumatoid Arthritis and Osteoarthritis. Glucosamine appears to help regenerate cartilage while the chondritin inhibits the enzymes that breakdown cartilage.

A combination pill of these two agents along with the addition of some anti-inflammatory herbs such as tumeric, sea cucumber, boswella, bromelain and "fever few" would appear to be an ideal product for arthritic joints.

CETYL MYRISTOLEATE (CM): Cetyl myristoleate is a medium chain fatty acid similar to flax oil, borage oil, evening primrose oil, and fish oil.

The primary work on this fascinating substance was performed by Dr. Harry Diehl at the National Institute of Health. Dr. Diehl discovered that Freund's adjuvant (heat- killed mycobacterium butyricum) which was being used to cause an arthritis in rats *failed to cause arthritis in Swiss albino mice.* These mice had cetyl myristoleate (CM), which protected them from the Freund's adjuvant arthritis. *When CM was injected into rats before the Freund's adjuvant they did not develop arthritis.*

Later, Dr. Diehl developed moderately severe osteoarthritis, so he gave himself CM. *In a few weeks he was free of joint symptoms and his chronic headaches had disappeared along with his chronic bronchitis.* This led to treating his daughter's chronic back pain and pains in 500 friends and relatives with CM. *Nearly all became symptom free and have remained so for 10 years. Persons who are going to respond to CM will start to improve in the first weeks and progress to complete recovery in 30 days. They generally do not need to take more CM.*

It appears that CM is 98% effective against both rheumatoid arthritis and osteoarthritis. This means that the arthritis is either cured or greatly improved. Benefits are reported in the following conditions:

Chronic foot and ankle pains may get rapid total improvement.

Temporomandibular joint (TMJ) and carpal tunnel syndrome (CTS) are often alleviated. TMJ is a huge problem for many patients. There is no clearly curative treatment.

Operations attempted for TMJ have not relieved the intractable pain and the patient is often left with worse pain after the surgery. An appliance to correctly position the mandible may help some persons. *Any therapy that can stop this problem is very welcome.*

Carpal tunnel syndrome is a very common problem, which results in loss of work and may need surgery that is not always curative. An effective way of treating CTS would also be a great blessing

Sports injuries complicated by lingering pain are often cured.

Emphysema and similar lung disorders improve dramatically. The scar tissue remains but the volume of inspired air may increase by up to 35%. Progression of the illness is stopped. There are no known medical treatments that change emphysema by a significant degree and the usual course is steady loss of lung function, with a fatal outcome.

Diabetics experience a lowering of insulin dosage and in some cases insulin was able to be discontinued.

CM appears to improve memory and increase energy.

Blood pressure improves in many patients.

Inflammatory illnesses such as ulcerative colitis and Crohn's Disease are significantly improved. This is very welcome news, *as both these diseases are often very difficult to treat.*

Some cases of psoriasis and eczema appear to improve.

In another study, 48 persons who had rheumatoid arthritis, osteoarthritis, or a reactive arthritis (Reiter's Syndrome, Psoriatic Arthritis, Arthritis following shigella, yersinia, salmonella, and campylobacter infections, and ankylosing spondylitis) were treated with CM.

These patients varied from mild to crippled. Two patients showed less than a 75% return of joint mobility. *The remaining 46 persons had from 80% to 100% return of joint movement and from 70% to 100% decrease in pain. Some patients even experienced partial correction of deformities.*

The fascinating thing about CM is that most patients have permanent benefits after 30 days of therapy(2 pills three times daily).

The improvement in emphysema is very important, as there is no other treatment that improves this disease. As with many other natural health treatments, there are no known side effects.

CETYL MYRISTOLATE can be obtained from Brower Enterprises 800-373 6076 and from *Natural Health Team* 800-416-2806.

MSM

Metylsulfonylmethane(MSM) in a dosage of 1000 mg. daily is equal in efficacy to non steroidal anti-inflammatory therapy and is safer. This is available in health food stores.

CAPSAICIN

Capsaicin depletes the body of substance P, which is a neuropeptide that carries pain sensation. Ointments are clearly beneficial when used on painful joints. This can be found in health food stores.

Prolotherapy For Severe Back Pain

An old established treatment for chronic, severe back pain is called prolotherapy. This therapy is based on the idea that much disabling back pain is caused by weak ligaments and tendons. When these ligaments and tendons become weak the bones, muscles, and joints are able to move out of their correct position, producing pain. A sclerosing solution is injected into a painful site. The resulting inflammatory reaction stimulates the body to produce collagen fibers at the site and the ligaments become pulled into their proper position, with disappearance of the pain. Weekly injections may be needed for several months. Call the American Association of Osteopathic Medicine at 800 992 2063 to find a doctor who can do this for you.

Magnet Therapy

No one knows how magnets work but there appears to be no doubt that they are an effective way to relieve a chronic localized pain. They must *not* be used on a patient with cancer and they may interfere with proper pacemaker function and perhaps insulin pumps.

Fibromyalgia

Fibromyalgia (FM) is a common disease of unknown cause characterized by severe pain in tender points, which are very painful with pressure. This is associated with fatigue, insomnia, headaches (50%), and depression. A rheumatologist at a medical school told me a fascinating story about a patient with fibromyalgia who entered the hospital with a heart attack. Morphine cleared the chest pain, *but did nothing for the fibromyalgia pain.*

Decreased bone density found in some patients with fibromyalgia suggests that *some of these patients may actually be suffering from Vitamin D deficiency, which is a commonly under-diagnosed disease.* Obtaining a blood Vitamin D level will clarify this issue and therapy with calcium and vitamin D will be curative.

Immunocal

Immunocal is a milk-serum-protein concentrate that can raise cellular glutathione (GTH). Glutathione is a powerful free radical scavenger. GTH is composed of three amino acids (glutamine, cysteine, and glycine). Immunocal has shown some fascinating clinical results.

Bill Cooper, 47 years old, developed stage 4 cancer of the larynx. Following surgery, radiation and chemotherapy he suffered nausea and was unable to eat, with subsequent 65-pound weight loss. Two weeks after being started on immunocal his nausea ceased and he began to gain weight.

Eva Beames took 20 tylenol tablets (acetaminophen AMP) daily for her fibromyalgia. She spent a fortune seeking help and finally tried Immunocal. Four days later, her energy came back and she began to work in her garden. Ten days later she realized *that all her back, leg, and ankle pain was gone.*

Perhaps acetaminophen, which is known to be a potent generator of free radicals and an agent that lowers glutathione levels in the liver, was contributing to her fibromyalgia.

Paula Rettig is another patient with fibromyalgia. She found 70% relief from her pain 2 weeks after starting Immunocal .

These two patients raise the interesting possibility that deficiency of GTH might be playing a role in this illness. Vitamin D lack is also a possible cause for these symptoms.

Henry Cheang developed early stage full lens cataracts. Four months later he began Immunocal. His cataracts slowly dissolved.

The lens has long been known to be depleted of glutathione when a cataract has developed. For patients with fibromyalgia who fail to respond to Immunocal, some symptomatic therapy can be helpful.

Low serotonin levels in patients with fibromyalgia may be helped by 5 hydroxytryptophane (5HTP) which treats depression. A dosage of 100 mg. three times daily helped 50% of patients get relief from pain, fatigue, and insomnia.

Sleep studies of fibromyalgia have shown that the patients have very little stage 4 sleep, which is the most restful and restorative stage of sleep. Melatonin may help with sleep and boosts growth hormone levels.

In 1999 a study published in PAIN showed patients with fibromyalgia have dihydroepiandosterone (DHEA) levels that are much lower than age - matched control groups. Furthermore, the lower the level of DHEA the worse the pain was. DHEA may be beneficial.

One third of the patients with FM have low levels of insulin growth factor, suggesting a possible low level of growth hormone. In 1998, a study where daily doses of growth hormone were injected revealed improvement after 6 months. *See our website for an effective new therapy for fibromyalgia. This uses thymic extract, bromelain, natural progesterone, and growth hormone with progressive resistance exercise.*

Relaxin Therapy

Relaxin is a hormone that relaxes the pubic ligaments during pregnancy and prepares the pelvis for delivery. Dr. Samuel Yue noted that his female fibromyalgia patients *were free of symptoms during pregnancy.* He then began to treat his fibromyalgia patients with relaxin over a 10 week time frame. with good results.

An interesting side effect of this therapy is the discovery that relaxin treatment seems to reverse aging skin damage, repairs skin injured by sunlight, accelerates wound healing, promotes the synthesis of collagen fibrils, and may prove beneficial in patients with scleroderma. Relaxin can be obtained as *Vitalexin* from Smart Basics 800-878 6520

Chronic Fatigue Syndrome (CFS)

Chronic fatigue syndrome is a condition that leaves it's victims with prolonged fatigue, headaches, and trouble sleeping. The disease in some patients appears to be caused by a virus. Patients with this entity complain of fatigue, headaches, and poor sleeping.

Aspartic acid is a key component in the Kreb's cycle, which permits the body to obtain energy from carbohydrates. European researchers in the 1950's observed that a compound composed of magnesium and potassium combined with a non essential amino acid asparate (aspartic acid) had some interesting properties:

The thymus gland of animals was protected from radiation damage by Magnesium Potassium Aspartate

(MPA).

Animals pretreated with MPA survived longer and radiation damage was more rapidly repaired than in controls.

Physical endurance seemed to be markedly increased with MPA.

MPA works in humans as well. Ninety per cent of patients experiencing post surgical fatigue that lasted more than one year were cured by MPA. Some felt well in three days while others needed two weeks. The dosage of MPA was 1 gram twice daily.

Subsequent studies have confirmed that 75% to 94% of fatigue plagued patients are helped by MPA. Many persons taking MPA can stop this therapy when their fatigue is gone. Others,however, need to continue taking it in a reduced dosage. Since fatigue plays such a prominent role in Chronic Fatigue Syndrome, a trial of MPA should be a good idea.

Make sure you order potassium magnesium aspartate, because oxides, chlorides, and gluconates will not work. This product can be obtained from *For Your Health Pharmacy* 800-888 4585

Systematic Lupus Erythematosis (SLE)

This disease is an auto- immune illness in which the body appears to be attacking itself. The disease involves collagen tissue in skin, joints, and the lining membranes over the lungs, heart, and abdomen. Occasionally, the kidneys and brain are seriously affected. SLE can often be markedly helped by thymic extract (see Chapter 3 IMMUNE ILLNESSES) Another approach that appears to have merit is use of DHEA (Dihydroepiandosterone).

DHEA Lupus is a disease mainly afflicting women. Flareups often occur premenstrually or during pregnancy.

Studies from Japan have revealed that women with lupus have very low levels of DHEA and low amounts of interleukin 2. Supplemental DHEA has increased interleukin 2 levels and has a dramatic benefit in symptoms.

Studies with Dr. van Vollenhoven at Stanford Medical School have confirmed the benefits of DHEA .The doses of prednisone in these patients were able to be decreased by 50% after taking DHEA. Usually 100 mg. of DHEA was needed to bring DHEA into high normal blood levels.

Scleroderma

Scleroderma is a chronic disease, which is characterized by skin thickening and scarring. The disease can be fatal if it involves the lungs, kidneys, joints, gastrointestinal tract and heart. The cardinal feature of the illness is extensive scarring of the involved tissues. The cause is unknown and there is no clear curative treatment.

DMSO (dimethyl sulfoxide) is a good treatment for Scleroderma. This can be used orally, intravenously or topically. Topical usage seems to be preferred on stiff swollen painful joints. In severe cases this can be given intravenously.

DMSO is a very valuable asset for the trainers of professional football teams and racing horses, where it permits rapid reversal of traumatic injuries.

DMSO can be obtained from DMSO Marketing 800-367 6935

GAMMA-LINOLENIC ACID is an essential fatty acid found in borage oil, evening primrose oil, or black current seed oil. These substances decrease the number of attacks of Raynaud's Syndrome, which may occur in scleroderma. In Raynaud's Syndrome, the small blood vessels of the hands, feet, ears, and nose go into spasm. The resulting pallor and white discoloration can be very painful.

Borage oil and evening primrose oil can be found in health food stores.

Chapter 7

Is There Any Safe Way To Improve Muscle Endurance?

Many athletes are anxious to be stronger and able to perform longer. Previous attempts to accomplish this with high doses of synthetic androgens have caused grave health problems, including liver damage, heart attacks, high blood cholesterol and triglyceride levels, androgen rage and atrophy of the testes.

In 1968 a renowned physiologist, Bjorn Ahlborg, demonstrated that 5 grams of Potassium Magnesium Aspartate given in divided dosage, with one dose given one hour before exercise, could increase the endurance of well trained athletes by 50% on a maximum stress test.

The athletes pedaled a stationary bike to a heart rate of 170 then continued until exhaustion or leg pain caused them to stop. *The athletes receiving MPA were able to continue for 128 minutes, while those not receiving MPA had to quit at 85 minutes.* The MPA appeared to increase the regeneration of ATP and improve the flow of electrolytes across the muscle cell membranes. Dr. Ahlborg used 1.75 grams four times daily in his study.

Competitive athletes might take 3 tablets of MPA three times daily with another three tablets one hour before the athletic event. The product is natural and has no known side effects. This can be obtained from *For Your Life Health Pharmacy* 800-888 4585

A second way to improve athletic performance appears to be obtainable from a form of ZMAX. ZMAX is an anabolic mineral complex containing a patented form of zinc 1-monomethionine, zinc magnesium aspartate and Vitamin B 6. Magnesium aids in the transport of oxygen to muscles and activates enzymes needed for carbohydrate and protein metabolism. Zinc aids in overcoming fatigue by minimizing the buildup of lactic acid in muscle tissue. Zinc also is required for the production of growth hormone and testosterone.

College football players took either a placebo or ZMAX, three tablets nightly for three weeks. Those receiving the ZMAX experienced the following benefits:

- 15% higher magnesium levels

- 33% higher zinc levels

- 43% higher total testosterone levels

- 44% higher free testosterone levels

- 25% higher Insulin-like Growth Factor (IGF-1)

- 2.5 fold increase in muscle strength

Increased physical endurance, rate of healing, mental alertness, and restful sleep were also observed. Decreased muscle cramps, strains, and water retention were also noted.

By aiding absorption and availability of zinc and magnesium, ZMAX safely raises testosterone levels in both men and women.

Because maximal healing and tissue repair occur about 90 minutes after sleep, when growth hormone is released from the pituitary gland, this treatment is given 30 to 60 minutes before sleep. The dosage is three capsules for men and two for women.

This natural product can be obtained from Smart Basics, Inc. 800-878-6520

Chapter 8

Osteoporosis

Osteoporosis is a disease in which profound softening of the bones leads to great disability with fractures often involving the hips and vertebra. This condition is very common in elderly women and persons who have taken cortisone for long periods of time. Hip fractures may actually *precede* the fall to the ground, as the bone is so fragile it breaks while the person is standing.

Countries that depend on vegetables for calcium intake have far fewer cases of osteoporosis than countries where large amounts of dairy products are consumed, as is the custom in the U.S.A.

Factors that contribute to osteoporosis are:

Excessive Intake of Phosphorus

The correct ratio of phosphorus to calcium intake is 1 to 1 .The average American has a skewed ratio of between 2 to 4 to 1. This ratio is disturbed because of the large intake of sodas (very high in phosphorus) and junk food. The body tries to correct for this disparity by breaking down bone to release calcium and restore the ratio toward 1 to 1.This injures bone.

Sedentary Lifestyle

Bones that are not being used develop softening with loss of calcium. This *always* appears in the bone that is immobilized in a cast. *Bones that are involved in physical activity become stronger*. Nature does not build bone that is not being used. Osteoporosis is rare in persons doing hard manual labor.

High Protein Diet

The average American consumes 100 grams of protein daily, instead of the desired 40 to 50 grams. That's double what they should consume. In a large population study, 1600 women who ate a vegetarian diet lost 18% of their bone by age 80, *whereas women who were meat eaters had lost 35% of their bone by age 80.* In the metabolism of protein, acid is produced which must be neutralized by calcium and magnesium leached from bone.

Excess Alcohol Consumption

Alcohol consumption in excess of a few ounces daily interferes with calcium absorption. 31% of males below the age of 40 who drank heavily had osteoporosis. *This is a devastating per cent,* because men are less prone to osteoporosis than women and osteoporosis is far more common in older individuals.

Excessive Consumption of Coffee

There is a 300% increase in the number of hip fractures, when you compare the greatest consumers of coffee with those who consume the least.

Overly Vigorous Exercise

Excessive exertion inhibits bone growth and gives rise to stress fractures. There is calcium loss during strenuous exercise.

Cigarette Smoking

Cigarette smoking inhibits calcium absorption, increases calcium loss, and interferes with the proper rebuilding of bone. Patients with broken bones need to quit smoking to permit bone healing.

Deficiency of Vitamin D

Vitamin D is present only in foods where it is added. It must be taken as a supplement, or the natural way, from the sun. *Twenty to forty minutes a day in the sun would produce adequate amounts of vitamin D*, but the use of sun- screens makes this of no value. A 1998 study in the New England Journal of Medicine showed that of 290 consecutive admissions to a general wards, 57% of patients were deficient in vitamin D blood levels. 42% of those below 65 years were also found to be deficient in vitamin D.

Drugs May Impair Calcium Metabolism

Cortisone, anti-convulsants, aluminum antacids, diuretics, tetracycline, lithium, anticoagulants, and phenothiazines can increase bone loss.

Excessive Consumption of Dairy Products.

Milk products, because they are so rich in protein, *often cause greater calcium loss than gain,* i.e. negative calcium balance, when taken in excessive amounts.

Birth Control Pills

These pills produce folic acid deficiency. Where there is a lack of folic acid homocysteine blood levels rise and this is associated with osteoporosis.

Excessive Salt Intake

When too much salt is taken in, there is an increase in calcium loss in the urine.

Fluoride produces abnormal bone, which is more likely to break.

Osteoporex

Osteoporex was developed by Dr.Brazzach, at the University of Sao Paolo, Brazil. Dr. Brazzach found an algae off the coast of Chile that contained calcium that could be 90% absorbed. (Calcium carbonate is only 8% absorbed.)

Dr. Brazzach then discovered that if he added vitamin D3 from shark cartilage, this greatly increased the effectiveness of the algae to heal osteoporotic bone.

The next step was to add Zedoary to the product. This is a powerful anti-inflammatory plant. This increased the effect of the product. Lastly, they added panax ginseng to the product. The reasoning behind this last addition was that hormone therapy is beneficial to osteoporosis and this compound has a hormone- like chemical structure. *The final formulation is so effective that in 95% of patients the bone density is restored by 4%, within 6 months.* Subsequently, the treatment needs to be used only 3 months each year. The 5% who failed to benefit all had cancer. 90% of the ingested algae calcium is absorbed.

Osteoporex has been renamed OsteoOrganiCAL and can be obtained from Natural Option Corporation 800-516 9796

Natural Progesterone Therapy For Osteoporosis

Dr. John Lee of Sebastapol, California has developed a natural program for treating osteoporosis that has produced striking improvements in bone density.

Patients were placed on a diet rich in green vegetables with low fat cheese. Red meat was limited to three times weekly. All sodas were eliminated, as the high phosphorus content interferes with calcium absorption. Alcohol use was minimized and cigarettes were forbidden.

Supplementation with the following was given:

- Calcium -- 800 to 1000 mg. daily

- Vitamin D -- 400 units daily

- Vitamin C -- 2000 mg in divided doses

- Beta Carotene -- 15 mg daily

Exercise was encouraged 20 minutes daily or 30 minutes three times weekly. Bone grows only when stress is applied to it (exercise).

Patients who were on estrogen continued to take .3 to .625 mg of conjugated estrogen (Premarin) for three weeks each month.

Patients applied a cream containing 3% natural progesterone (Fem-Gest) at bedtime daily, for twelve days each month. For those taking estrogen, the cream was to be applied the last two weeks of the month. Between one third and one half of a one ounce jar of progesterone was to be applied each month. The Fem-Gest Cream may be applied to the neck, breast, face, or abdomen.

Dr. Lee's study involved 100 women and lasted three years. Most patients had already lost height, some as much as 5 inches. By adding the progesterone cream, the bone density could be increased as much as 10% in the first 6 months and then increased annually at a rate of 3 to 5% annually.

Two surprising results of the study were that neither age or time from menopause had any influence on the restoration of bone. In fact the persons with the lowest bone densities had the fastest increases. *The bone density tests showed steady improvement until the density was that of a healthy 35 years old.* There were no pathological fractures in these women. No side effects were seen. Lancet 90; 336[8726] : 1327

Estrogen acts on the osteoclast and stops further loss of bone. Natural progesterone acts on the osteoblast cells to increase the formation of new bone. *Natural progesterone leads to the creation of new bone and complete reversal of osteoporosis.* All persons living in developed countries are estrogen dominant by virtue of exposure to xenoestrogens, which are primarily petrochemical in origin.

Because progesterone levels go to nothing after menopause and estrogen levels persist at approximately 40% of normal by virtue of continued estrogen production from fat tissue, adrenal glands and the ovary, the further use of estrogen compounds the already existing problem of estrogen dominance. For these reasons the rational therapy for osteoporosis is *natural progesterone*.

Violetto Chamarro, the former President of Nicaragua, was incapacitated by osteoporosis. Dr. David Williams gave her natural progesterone and in a few months she was dramatically improved.

Fem-Gest is obtained from Mexican yam and contains aloe vera, Vitamin E, and a vegetable base. Fem-Gest was initially formulated by Bio Nutritional Formulas Inc. They now make an identical product called *Dr.'s Pride Pure-Gest,* which has no preservatives.

Dr.'s Pride Pure-Gest can be obtained from 800- 950 –8484 or from our *Natural Health Team* 800-416-2806.

Chapter 9

Insomnia

Many persons suffer from poor sleeping. Melatonin is a hormone produced by the pineal gland that is responsive to light. When darkness begins, blood melatonin levels start to rise leading to sleep. Melatonin production declines as we age, which could explain why sleep problems are so common in the elderly.

Melatonin has exceptional antioxidant activity, being both fat and water soluble. This permits it to cross into and protect the brain from free radicals. Melatonin also boosts the immune system by facilitating the action of helper T cells, which coordinate the immune response. It directly attacks tumor cells and inhibits cancer growth.

Large doses (10 mg. to 40 mg) have reduced tumor size and prolonged life in patients with cancer of breast, lung, colon, brain, and stomach.

There is animal based evidence suggesting that melatonin may prolong life. This remains to be seen.

Melatonin has proven to be *very* effective in improving sleep. It has also been of benefit in stopping jet lag after long airplane flights.

There is no problem with addiction and melatonin is safe. The usual dose is 3 mg but smaller doses may be effective.

Who Should Take Melatonin?

There are 3 reasons, other than sleep enhancement, that make melatonin a possible benefit to many:

1. As an antioxidant it protects the brain, cardiovascular system and other systems from free radical damage.

2. By boosting the immune system melatonin guards against cancer and infectious diseases.

3. Melatonin has a regulatory function in the endocrine system, which boosts the production of growth hormone, *the most effective anti-aging substance yet known.*

Melatonin can be obtained in health food stores and from *Natural Health Team* 800-416-2806..

Topical application of essential oils (rose, lavender or ylang ylang) by rubbing up and down the spine at bedtime, calm, relax and usually result in a restful night of sleep.

Chapter 10

HIV Infection

HIV infections are associated with profound injury to the immune system. In this state of severe inability to prevent infections, one serious infection after another may occur.

One treatment has been beneficial to an HIV patient is thymic extract. This was discussed extensively in Chapter 2 Immune Illnesses.

Hepatitis C is a very serious, potentially fatal viral illness. With thymic extract treatment, the symptoms may clear up and the blood serology tests for hepatitis C can return to normal. This suggests that thymic extract could work very well in the viral disease HIV as well.

A second agent that could benefit HIV disease is dimethyl glycine, which was discussed in Chapter 2 on Immune Illnesses.

A third agent that I would encourage in HIV problems is SBO (Soil Based Organisms). This has been reported to be beneficial in hepatitis B and C, chronic fatigue syndrome, AIDS and influenza. This will be discussed in much more detail in Chapter 17 on Gastrointestinal Diseases.

A fourth product that could be considered for use in HIV is *Immunocal*, which was discussed in Chapter 6 on Arthritis.

This compound seems to raise levels of glutathione, which could be helpful to an HIV patient where GTH is depressed.

Sterinol also appears to benefit HIV patients (see Chapter 6) on Rheumatoid Arthritis).

Padma has also stabilized patients with HIV infection.

Chapter 11

Impotence

There are two problems simultaneously occurring among males in the United States. The first of these is a steadily rising number of males who are having trouble with impotence. Additionally, population studies have shown that for the past 50 years there has been a continuous decline in sperm counts, sperm motility, and fertility in U.S. males. The reason for this is not certain but *widespread exposure to estrogen is the suspected culprit.*

Males and females in industrialized, developed nations (any country with lots of cars, trucks, and factories) are exposed to estrogen on a daily basis. *Environmental compounds called xenoestrogens, which are primarily of petrochemical origin, have very potent estrogen-like activity.* These are found in our air, fuels, pesticides, herbicides, plastics, clothing and personal care products such as propylene glycol and sodium laurel sulfate.

Male offspring born to *xenoestrogen-exposed parents often have a lowered sperm count.*

The food we eat is often *contaminated with hormones. Synthetic estrogen* is used to fatten cattle, chickens, and other meat-producing animals and to increase milk and egg production.

Men naturally have a small amount of progesterone in their body. This progesterone is converted directly to testosterone. *Men over the age of 45 may well find that the increase in testosterone resulting from natural progesterone will raise their testosterone levels, which can cause improved potency and libido and better muscle tone.* Males who have had either surgical castration or chemical castration as therapy for prostate cancer cannot be given testosterone but may safely supplement with natural progesterone. This *natural progesterone* will replace testosterone in promoting new bone growth and will not have feminizing effects.

Impotence is a common problem. Any condition that blocks the blood flow to the penis (arteriosclerosis, smoking, diabetes, hypertension, and high cholesterol) can be associated with impotence.

Impotence can also be caused by blood pressure medicines, antidepressants, drugs that block the secretion of acid from the stomach (zantac, tagamet), sedatives, painkillers, tranquilizers, and prostate therapy, pituitary tumor (prolactin secreting), aging with reduced testosterone production, and alcohol, marijuana, cocaine, and tobacco.

Seven therapeutic approaches will be discussed. The first of these is:

Growth Hormone

Many elderly males have reported improved sexual performance after starting therapy with growth hormone. This is a very physiologic way of restoring normal function of the hormones involved in a correct sexual response. Growth hormone will be discussed in more detail in Chapter 25 on LONGEVITY. This can be obtained from our *Natural Health Team*.

Arginine

Arginine is a non-essential amino acid that has a vital function as a precursor for Nitric Oxide (NO). *When arginine is given to an individual, that person will have higher levels of NO in their body.* NO acts as a messenger for many body functions. It signals the release of important hormones and functions as a neurotransmitter in the brain. The immune system uses *NO* to kill bacteria and cancer cells.

Adequate levels of *NO* keep the blood pressure normal, prevent heart disease, and maintain proper circulation.

Nitric oxide is a key to good erections. To have an erection, *NO* acting on a message from the brain triggers the release of a compound that relaxes the muscles in the spongy part of the penis, allowing it to fill with blood. If there is not enough *NO*, there will be no erection.

Arginine in a dose of 1.5 grams about 45 minutes before intercourse may lead to a firmer erection by raising *NO* levels. A regular dosage of 2 grams of arginine, three times daily may also prove beneficial. Because this approach deals with the fundamental cause for inadequate sexual performance (lack of needed *NO*) and because it is safe, I think arginine has merit.

Consult your physician if you take Viagra or nitroglycerine or if you have migraine, HIV, cirrhosis, depression, or cancer, before starting treatment. If there is no improvement in erections in two months, this should be stopped. Being a natural substance, it has no known harmful side effects.

Testosterone

As males age, their levels of testosterone slowly fall. If impotence appears, regular injections of testosterone can be helpful. It is important that the person be checked for prostate cancer before and during treatment, with PSA blood tests and regular rectal exams, because rising testosterone levels can trigger prostate cancer.

Muira Puama

Muira puama is a plant from Brazil. 1 to 1.5 grams of extracts of this plant used in 250 patients with impotence led to increased libido in 62% and improved erections in 51%. This can be obtained from Enzymatic Therapy 800-783 2286

Dihydroepiandosterone (DHEA)

This hormone is a precursor to the construction of many other hormones.

Levels of DHEA are maximal at age 20 and fall by 80% when an individual reaches 65. Rebuilding these levels with oral DHEA seems to reverse death rates in elderly males, possibly by blocking the production of fatty acids and cholesterol. There is a strong argument that *all* persons over 50 years should be taking this substance.

There is a real hope that DHEA can counteract stress, improve clarity of thought and memory, functions as an antioxidant and may help protect against cancer and osteoporosis. Dosage is 50 mg. daily in males and 25 mg. daily in females..

Individuals with impotence may experience rising testosterone blood levels that can help impotence. The same cautions about diagnosing prostate cancer are obviously needed.

Maca

Maca is from a plant found in the high parts of Peru. In a dosage of 500 mg daily this is reported to help erection problems. This can be obtained from health food stores.

ZMAX

ZMAX offers a different approach to the problem of impotence. This product raises the level of testosterone by 43%, while also increasing IGF-1 growth factor. Whether this would be adequate to improve potency *has not been studied*, but this may be a safe way to raise testosterone levels. More information about ZMAX was given in Chapter 7.

Natural Progesterone

Because of the xenoestrogen exposure that prevails in modern society, all males in developed nations are estrogen dominant. Therapy with natural progesterone will help correct this problem and appears to have helped many males with impotence. Progesterone is converted to testosterone in men and this can help with potency.

We like *Wild Yam Cream* as a safe, effective natural progesterone. The natural progesterone in this preparation is an extract of wild yams. The product also contains ginkgo biloba, damiana extract, gotu kola extract Siberian ginseng extract and saw palmetto. All these substances are believed to have beneficial effects on male sexual performance.

Apply one fourth to one half teaspoon to the skin of the inner thigh or inner arm daily. This is available from Advance Nutritional Products 888- 436 7200 and from our *Natural Health Team* 800-416-2806.

Chapter 12

Alcoholism

Dr. Roger Williams did experiments 40 years ago with alcohol that still have great interest. Some rats were fed 10% alcohol, others water. By simply adding or subtracting vitamins and minerals he could produce *or eliminate* alcoholism in the rats.

He discovered that the amino acid l-glutamine protects the body from the toxic effect of alcohol and *reduces alcohol cravings.*

An alcoholic woman was given tasteless l-glutamine in her food without her knowledge. Several weeks later she said, " I am going to stop drinking". She became employed and did not return to alcohol. Good nutrition can probably also help reduce alcohol cravings.

Alcoholics Anonymous

This wonderful organization has helped multitudes of alcoholics stay sober by use of a 12 step program based on Bible principles. I have known several severe alcoholics who ceased alcohol use after inviting Jesus Christ to become their personal savior. This same approach has worked well in helping persons with drug abuse(Narcotics Anonymous) and compulsive gambling(Gamblers Anonymous).

Several of my patients also were able to give up heavy use of cigarettes when Christ entered their lives.

Chapter 13

Overweight

There are more overweight people in the USA than in other nations. One reason for this might be the decrease in consumption of conjugated linoleic acid (CLA). CLA is vital for good health. It is found in beef, lamb, turkey and some milk products.

Human beings are unable to convert linoleic acid into the needed amount of *conjugated* linoleic acid. Decreased intake of conjugated linoleic acid and alterations in the manner of production and processing of the foods that contain CLA have led to overweight. Here's the problem: *if there is inadequate intake of CLA, dietary fat cannot be moved into cells or used as energy. The end result is that the body stores this fat. You get, and will remain, fat.*

The two primary sources of CLA are beef and milk, both of which are consumed much less than in previous generations because of concerns about saturated fat. This fact is compounded by the observation that the quantity of CLA in both beef and milk has been falling for 40 years. Milk has dropped from 3% to 1%. The reason for the fall in beef CLA is that cattle are being fattened on feedlots with feed instead of grazed, where they eat grass. Grazed cattle in Australia have meat with CLA levels *four times that of US beef.* Therefore, even increasing our intake of meat and milk may not accomplish very much.

CLA increases the metabolic rate in mice, allowing them to lose 43 to 88 per cent of their body fat in six weeks. The weight loss was associated with decreased appetite, which caused more fat cells to be used for energy production. These mice ended up with more muscle mass.

Human studies show that *CLA causes body fat in overweight individuals to go down by 20% in 12 weeks.* This fat loss occurs with intake of 3.4 grams of CLA daily. Higher doses of CLA did not lead to any greater weight loss. *This weight loss occurred without any changes in diet or exercise.*

Other studies in humans have revealed that CLA blocks the production of inflammatory cytokines that cause the destruction of joint cartilage. Additionally, CLA stops excess production of prostaglandin 2, which has been linked to both arthritis and osteoporosis.

Animals fed butterfat and CLA experienced less joint inflammation and were noted to have an increased rate of new bone formation. These human and animal experiments suggest that CLA may be beneficial to both arthritis and osteoporosis.

Animal studies have shown that CLA appears to prevent tumors from forming and, when they are present, their growth is stopped or slowed.

This information about CLA is further evidence that *good fat* has an essential role to play in human health. The major importance of essential fatty acid (Omega 3 deficiency) also shows how vital the intake of the *proper* fat is to our good health.

This evidence about CLA supports the concept that lack of the correct type of dietary fat can cause obesity.

Hyperinsulinemia also causes obesity. Overweight individuals are trapped with an inability to lose weight despite their best intentions to diet. Nothing will be accomplished until their conjugated linoleic acid levels or hyperinsulinemia are corrected, so that fat can be burned instead of stored.

Clearly, following a diet when you have too much insulin or not enough conjugated linoleic acid is destined for failure. Your best efforts to diet will not work. For the person who is in doubt which path to pursue, we would suggest first getting a blood insulin level. If this level is normal, then start CLA therapy. If the insulin level is high, get started on flax oil, stop consuming *synthetic* fats, and restrict your daily fat intake to less than 25% of total calories. Furthermore, lack of conjugated linoleic acid may be contributing to problems with both arthritis and osteoporosis.

The softgel contains 1000 mg of safflower oil, 750 mg of which is CLA. Therefore if you take 4 softgels daily you will get 3 grams of CLA daily, plus a small amount from your food.

This supplement can be obtained under the name *Tonalin* from *Mountain Home Nutritionals* at 800- 888 1415 and from *Natural Health Team* 800-416-2806.

Flax Oil

One beneficial effect seen in persons using flax oil is improved metabolism. Better metabolism often leads to weight loss in individuals taking flax oil. I personally use flax oil and my appetite is satisfied with smaller quantities of food than previously eaten.

Lipidox

This supplement contains l-carnitine, chromium picolate, pyruvate, and hydroxyveitrate. The first three optimize the liver's ability to burn fat and the hydroxyveitrate is an apetite suppressant.

In an article in Medical Hypothesis in 1999, 16 subjects were placed on a low fat diet along with 12 grams of calcium pyruvate, 1.5 grams of HCA, 250 mg of l-carnitine and 600 mg of chromium picolate along with daily aerobic exercise. The average weight loss in one month was 13.2 pounds. They lost 5 pounds of fat weekly and gained 1.76 pounds of muscle each week. Aerobic exercise must be performed to see good results from this therapy.

Chapter 14

Malignancies (Cancer, Lymphoma, Leukemia)

The survival rates for treatment of cancer are not much better than they were 25 years ago. The reason for this may lie in pursuing chemotherapy and radiation as the primary modes of therapy. Obviously, surgery when a cancer is localized is an effective therapy. Both chemotherapy and radiation damage the immune system.

Cancer is most probably caused by a failure of the immune system to detect and destroy a cell that has become malignant. Therefore, it is easy to understand why methods of therapy that injure the immune system (radiotherapy, chemotherapy) are not leading to improved survival.

The immune system can also be injured by alcohol, smoking and age. The effects of heavy use of both alcohol and cigarettes is well illustrated by the fact that cancers of the upper nasal passages are about *8 times more common* in these individuals than in non users of alcohol and cigarettes.

I believe that efforts to heal the immune system will be more likely to eventually lead to a cure for cancer than developing new chemotherapy agents.

Is there any evidence that this approach could work?

Yes. There is a multitude of data supporting this approach. Researchers at the University of Victoria in British Columbia did a careful follow up on 200 persons who underwent a "spontaneous remission of cancer".

They found that 87% of these persons had switched diets, usually to a vegetarian diet. This does not mean that everyone who goes on a vegetarian diet is going to recover from cancer. However, it certainly raises the possibility that what we eat might be a factor in why we got cancer and what we eat might also tip the scales toward recovery. High intake of saturated fat is known to be a risk factor for the development of lung, breast, colon, prostate cancer and lymphomas.

There is a brilliant researcher in Germany named Dr. Joanna Budwig, who was several times nominated for the Nobel Prize. About forty years ago, she discovered that all cancer patients were lacking key nutrients (linoleic acid, phosphatides, and albumin) in their blood. These nutrients were present in healthy blood and the lack of these nutrients had permitted the cancer cells to grow in an uncontrolled manner. When they recovered, these key nutrients had been restored.

She began to treat cancer cases with 2 tablespoons of flax oil and 4 tablespoons of cottage cheese (quark) twice daily. The cottage cheese supplied sulfur with protein and was critical to recovery, as the *flax oil alone would not correct the metabolic abnormality.* Dr. Budwig now has more than 1,000 cured cancer victims in her practice. *Many of these persons were nearly dead when she took over their care. Here is clear indication that correct food can contribute towards healing cancer.*

While there are no known cures for cancer, there are steps, which can be taken which may well help alleviate the disease.

Selenium

In a December 1996 article in the Journal of the American Medical Association, Dr. Larry Clark presented evidence that supplemental selenium could reduce cancer death rates by as much as 50%. 1,312 patients were given 200 mcg. of selenium daily. The patients receiving selenium had a rise of 67% in their blood selenium level.

The patients receiving selenium had a 67% decrease in cancer of the prostate, a 58 percent decrease in colon or rectal cancer and a 45% decrease in lung cancer. This suggests that possibly up to 100,000 lives a year might be saved in the USA *by the simple addition of selenium to the diet.*

Why Does This Happen?

Selenium is a powerful antioxidant which also generates the production of glutathione(GTH). GTH mops up hydrogen peroxide, a potent free radical, which is created in the body during normal metabolism.

Selenium facilitates quick repair of damage to the DNA molecule. This stops damaged DNA molecules from reproducing and thus helps prevent the initiation of a tumor.

It contributes towards the death of cancerous and pre-cancer cells. Their death appears to occur before they replicate, thus helping stop cancer before it gets started. This is a trace metal food supplement that appears to be able to prevent the development of cancer. Do not exceed the recommended dosage of 200 mcg daily, as selenium causes toxic effects in *excessively* high dosages.

Lycopene

47,894 health care workers were carefully tracked during a four- year test. None had prostate cancer at the beginning of the study but 773 had developed prostate cancer by the finish. Men who ate 10 servings a week of tomatoes and tomato sauce on pizzas had 45% less cancer of the prostate than those eating no tomatoes. Surprisingly, tomatoes on pizza seemed more beneficial than raw tomato, suggesting that heating the tomato paste increases the anticancer effect. This study confirms previous studies of Mediterreanean people, who showed that they had one of the lowest rates of prostate cancer. Afro-Americans eat few tomatoes and they had the highest rate of prostate cancer.

Vitamin E

In a study in the Journal of the National Cancer Institute, men taking vitamin E had 32% less prostate cancer and 41% fewer deaths from prostate cancer than another control group.

How Does Vitamin E Work?

Vitamin E is very active as an antioxidant in fatty tissues. It breaks up lipid peroxidation in the mitochondrial membranes and wards off the free radicals generated by heavy metals, toxins from the environment, drugs, and radiation. When hit by a free radical, it oxidizes but may still recover usefulness if there is adequate glutathione, vitamin C, coenzyme Q10, and lipoic acid in the vicinity.

The correct dose of Vitamin E appears to be 800 i.u. daily, preferably of *natural* origin.

Coenxzyme Q10

Dr. Per Langsjoen, a cardiologist, had a patient with a surgical diagnosis of inoperable adenocarcinoma of the stomach. He was started on 240 mg daily of Co Q10 for heart disease. Five years later a CAT scan of the abdomen showed no evidence of cancer. Consider taking large doses of CoQ, 10 from 300 to 600 mg daily.

Prostate Cancer

Dr. James Talcott at the Center For Outcomes Research at the Massachusetts General Hospital believes that more than 75% of men with prostate cancer need no therapy over the course of their illness. Autopsies on men over age 80 disclose that 80% have microscopic areas of cancer in the prostate. Yet, only 4% of those men will die of prostate cancer.

A survey by the Journal of the American Medical Association disclosed that *"specialists tend to recommend the therapy they deliver"*. This means that urologists will advise radical surgery for cancer and the radiologist will suggest radiation therapy.

Watchful waiting is probably the best course except for young men, Afro-Americans, and those with high Gleason scores, all of whom do have a greater risk of rapid demise. These patients may need more aggressive treatment (surgery or radiation).

If the PSA begins to rise, a Chinese herbal therapy (PC SPES) often proves effective in treating the cancer, which coincides with a falling PSA value. This also works on those who at first responded and then relapsed on hormone therapy. *Antineoplaston* from Dr.Burzynski's clinic in Houston has also cured some prostate cancer.

For prostate cancer management, stay on a low fat diet, eat tomato products often, take a multivitamin, vitamins C, E and selenium.

If I developed prostrate cancer I would take flax oil and cottage cheese.

Chemotherapy And Radiation Therapy For Malignancies

Chemotherapy injures the bone marrow, which is the source of our immune cells. Remission occurs in *only 7%* of cases and prolonged survival in *only 15%.* The results of chemotherapy have to be considered dismal. Radiation is also injurious to the bone marrow.

What should you do if you have cancer?

An individual is primarily responsible for his own health. If you go to a poor physician and receive bad advice and follow it, *you will be the one who will suffer*. The MD may say, "I'm sorry", but *you* will suffer. When you go to a physician for advice about management of your cancer, you have every right to ask the following questions:

Will chemotherapy cure me?

Are there serious side effects from the chemotherapy treatment you propose?

If the answer to the first question is no or if the answer to the second question is yes, why jeopardize your life when there are safe, natural treatments which may prove helpful?

If you are on chemotherapy treatments or radiation and your white count gets depressed, you can develop a blood stream infection with pseudomonas, staphloccocus or enterococcus and die within two or three days.

I remember very well my thoughts when one of my patients was diagnosed with cancer. There was always a sickening feeling in my stomach when the time came to refer the patient for chemotherapy. Often the patient was well, but it was certain that he or she would be very sick in a few weeks from the chemotherapy. *And for what purpose?* They were going to die from cancer after being made very sick from the chemotherapy treatment. What a tragic way to leave this earth.

What are the alternatives to radiation and chemotherapy?

My suggestion is that flax oil and cottage cheese be the cornerstone of efforts to manage and deal with cancer for the following reasons:

We know that this treatment has benefited more than a thousand patients in the practice of Dr. Joanna Budwig.

Dr. Budwig has been unable to get papers about her cancer results published in medical journals, probably because one such paper might seriously damage sales of both chemotherapy drugs and artificial oils. For many years, Mr. Clifford Beckwith has provided cancer victims with an audiocassette telling of his remission of Stage 4 (advanced) cancer of the prostate by flax oil and cottage cheese.

His PSA fell from 75 to .1 after 6 months of flax oil. In the course of giving these audiotapes to many cancer victims he knew of more than 60 survivors in 1998 who took flax oil and cottage cheese.

Mr. Beckwith's cousin lost a wife to cancer. He is in contact with a group in Spain who have seen more than 90% of cancer victims who took cottage cheese and flax oil recover.

Dr. Budwig suggests thorough mixing of the cottage cheese with the flax oil. 4 tablespoons of flax oil could be mixed with 1 cup of cottage cheese and placed in a refrigerator. Eat all of this daily. If you are using high lignin flax oil, which appears desirable in treating malignancies, the lignans tend to settle in the bottom of the bottle. Bruce Barlean suggests vigorous shaking for 20 seconds before pouring to disperse the lignans. Pure fruit could be added such as strawberries or chopped apples, blueberries and pineapple.

Use only plain yogurt, not flavored and use twice as much yogurt as you would cottage cheese if you substitute yogurt for cottage cheese. Tofu also works in the same dosage as natural yogurt.

There is another way to take flax that should only be used in a desperate situation, as we cannot be sure that it works in cancer cases. If someone is nauseated by the oil, flax seed can be ground with a coffee grinder. Operate the grinder for about 13 to 15 seconds. This creates chaff that can be sprinkled into natural yogurt. Then chopped apples, bananas, strawberries, mangos, or blueberries can be added to create a delicious food. You can grind 8 tablespoons of flaxseed, which is equivalent to 4 tablespoons of flax oil. If more than one day's needs are ground, keep the remainder in a refrigerator until used. Probably no more than two or three days supply should be ground at one time.

Flax oil should be cold processed and unrefined. Cold processing means that the flax seed was pressed at temperatures below 110 degrees F.

When recovery has occurred, Dr. Budwig suggests reducing the flax oil dose to 1 tablespoon per 100 pounds of weight daily as maintenance, along with cottage cheese.

All flax oil is good if it has been not been refined and was *cold pressed* and kept refrigerated. *Flax oil lasts one year if frozen, four months if refrigerated and several months at room temperature.*

One woman with such advanced cancer she could not eat *was given flax oil and skimmed milk by enemas. Three months later, though not cured, she was well and able to care for her large family.*

In the cases that did not recover from cancer, they did not use enough flax oil in the beginning (4 oz. needed) or they switched to flax flakes. *The nutrient quality of flax is destroyed by heat so it is easy to comprehend why the flakes do not work, as there must be high temperatures involved in the manufacture of flakes.*

Flax capsules appear to be a menace as well, since several patients died after doing well on the oil when they switched to capsules. This means that flax should be taken as either flax seed (ground) or flax oil.

Several patients relapsed when they stopped flax oil after doing well. Probably, whatever caused them to get cancer was still present when they stopped flax oil. This therapy needs to be continued the rest of your life.

Several patients in Beckwith's study were clearly improving with flax oil when the MD insisted on more chemo. Sadly, these patients died after the new chemo shot. The results appeared poorer when chemo was being used at the same time as flax oil, *probably because the chemo was damaging what the flax oil was trying to build up.*

One patient gave me a chuckle. This patient with advanced pancreatic cancer was terminal in a Tennessee hospital when he started on flax oil.

This form of cancer is more than 99% fatal. After starting on flax oil he returned to his oncologist for an examination. The oncologist was so surprised at the recovery he said, *"we must have made a mistaken diagnosis"*. One of the 62 recovered patients had leukemia.

Mr. Beckwith has very graciously advised me that he would be delighted to provide his audio tape to any cancer victim who wanted to learn more about flax oil and cottage cheese. I think for anyone contemplating the use of this therapy it could be comforting to know that others are doing the same thing. You can contact Mr. Beckwith by email at spinner@usit.net

Summation: Why do I prefer flax oil for patients with cancer?

This has proved helpful to more than one thousand patients with cancer in Dr. Budwig's practice.

Would you give it to any member of my family with cancer?

The answer is yes. Here's why: this treatment often works and is safe. Furthermore, it is not expensive.

Perilla Oil

There are a few persons who do not tolerate flax oil. I am aware of a woman who developed a severe facial dermatitis after taking flax oil. Another woman became miserable with gaseous distress and continuous belching. For these persons there may be an effective alternative in Perilla Oil.

Perilla oil is derived from the beefsteak plant common in East Asia. *The oil from this plant is 50% pure alpha linolenic acid (Omega 3 Fatty acid)*. Perilla oil is active in blocking platelet-activating factor, which helps prevent blood clots. It has been known to lower cholesterol within 7 days in some patients.

Animal experiments in Japan have shown an effect against cancer. An intriguing piece of research in Japan revealed that rats fed either perilla oil or safflower oil had striking differences in their neurone development. *The rats on safflower oil, by the second generation performed poorly in learning new information when compared to the rats given perilla oil.*

These rats fed safflower *had 30% less neurone connections in their brains than the perilla fed rats. This suggests that dietary fat intake may have a major impact on brain development and intelligence.*

Perilla oil is less expensive than flax oil and might be a satisfactory therapy for the person unable to tolerate flax oil in cases of cancer. Perilla oil is sold in 1000 mg capsules, each containing 550 mg of alpha linolenic acid oil. Be sure to use cottage cheese, unflavored yogurt or tofu as directed for flax oil, because the protein which contains sulfur must be present to deal with the metabolic abnormality of malignancy. The dose is 3-6 capsules daily.

Perilla oil is available from Health–n-Energy 800-571 2999

Essiac

Essiac formula was given to nurse Rene Caisse more than 80 years ago by a woman whose breast cancer had been healed by this Ojibway Indian herbal preparation. The formula is composed of four herbs (burdock root, slippery elm, sheep sorrel, and Indian rhubarb). The burdock root contains inulin, which improves the function of white blood cells. This root also contains Vitamin A and selenium, which scavenge free radicals and chromium which regulates blood sugar levels.

Slippery elm has mucilage that benefits plasma and lymph. Sheep sorrel contains vitamins and trace minerals as well as silicon, which protect nerves. Indian rhubarb root has antibiotic and anti-tumor properties.

There is a long history of benefits in treating malignancies with *Essiac*.

A young male developed Hodgekin's Disease and began chemotherapy. After 5 treatments, he ran away from home to escape chemotherapy. Someone started him on *Essiac* and he made a complete recovery.

A Calgary Businessman began chemotherapy and radiation treatments for cancer of the prostate gland. He deteriorated and became a complete invalid. He was started on *Essiac* and eventually recovered.

Another male had nine operations to remove malignant bladder tumors. His recovery was believed to be unlikely until he was started on ESSIAC. After the *Essiac* he passed 40 pieces of malignant tissue in his urine and then made a complete recovery.

Another male developed small cell carcinoma of the lung and was given a 6 month life expectancy. A daughter urged him to try *Essiac*. The lung tumor disappeared and he became well.

A male developed inoperable lung cancer. He started *Essiac* and began to improve. Surgery was done to remove lymph nodes and what was felt to be residual cancer in the right lung. The pathology report disclosed no sign of tumor in either lung tissue or lymph nodes.

A male began *Essiac* for early colon cancer and the cancer disappeared.

In Reese Dubin's superb book, *Miracle Food Cures From The Bible,* (a study of medicinal foods used in the Bible) there are 33 pages about Essiac, which convincingly documents probable recovery from a wide variety of malignancies.

The correct way to take Essiac is as follows: Take two fluid ounces twice daily for one week. Take two fluid ounces three times daily for one week. Take 3 fluid ounces three times daily thereafter. Be sure to carefully follow the instructions about preparing the tea. We recommend you obtain this product from Resperin of Canada 888 - 900 2299 or from our *Natural Health Team* 1-800-416-2806.

MGN-3

Dr. Mamdooh Ghoneum developed a superb natural cancer treatment product in Japan. This is a combination of 3 mushrooms and rice bran. This combination appears to have a powerful beneficial effect on the immune system.

Natural killer cells (NK) are the first line defense of the body. They attach to a cancer cell and proceed to inject granules into the cancer cell, which cause it to explode, leading to cell death within 5 minutes.

When these NK cells neither recognize nor destroy the invader, the situation is serious. This may be the problem in cancer as well as AIDS patients. Dr.Ghoneum's work has shown that in 80 to 90% of cancer patients the killer cells kill onlyabout 20 to 30% of the cancer cells in the first hour of testing.

After two weeks of MGN-3 the kill percentage goes up to 60 to 70% of cancer cells in 99% of patients. This kill percentage continues to rise the longer therapy with MGN-3 is continued, so that after two months treatment they are killing 27 times more cancer cells than before therapy started. (International Journal of Immunotherapy 98:14 (2): 89-99).

Mgn-3 also increases the production of tumor necrosis factor. These are proteins that help destroy tumor cells.

Results:

Prostate Cancer: 2 complete remissions out of 3 patients.

Ovarian Cancer: 2 complete remissions out of 3 patients (this form of cancer has been hard to cure).

Breast Cancer: Complete remission 1 of 3. Partial remission in the other two

Multiple Myeloma: This is a malignancy of the plasma cell. *It has never been cured with chemotherapy.* Dr. Ghoneum treated one patient who was diagnosed and treated with chemotherapy. His symptoms cleared, but he still had a blood marker showing persistence of the disease. MGN 3 was started and 6 months later the blood tests were normal. *After 9 years he remains well, representing the first patient ever cured of multiple myeloma.*

Take four 250 mg. pills three times daily before meals for a period of two weeks. Then reduce the dosage to two 250mg. pills before breakfast and evening meal. This is the maintenance dosage.

This is available from CompassionNet 800- 510 2010 and our *Natural Health Team* 800-416-2806.

AHCC

This compound seems similar to MGN 3, as it is derived from mushrooms without rice bran. The substance is very active in improving immune function. NK (killer lymphocytes) have a 300% increase in activity similar to MGN 3

Another valuable property of AHCC is the ability to increase the formation of TNF (tumor necrosis factor). TNF are a group of proteins that destroy cancer cells.

AHCC has proven effective in treating patients with primary liver cancer (hepatoma) and patients whose cancer had originated elsewhere and had spread into the liver. The survival rates for hepatomas is only 3% to 5%, which occurs generally from successful surgical removal of a lobe of liver containing a mass of hepatoma.

In a study, 121 patients with hepatomas were divided into three groups:

A. These patients were started on AHCC immediately after surgery. (38 patients)

B. This group began AHCC if a recurrence of the hepatoma was discovered. (18 patients)

C. These patients were given a placebo. (65 patients).

After 3 to 4 years the survival rate was much higher in Group A than the other groups. Not only did more Group A patients survive longer *but many remained entirely free of cancer. This suggests a good response to AHCC.*

In Japan, more than 100,000 patients with cancer have been treated with AHCC. 60% showed some benefit with many appearing to go into remission.

Patients with cancer were treated with 1 gram of AHCC three times daily for three weeks then the dose was reduced to 500 mg twice daily.

AHCC can be obtained from Harmony Co. 800-404 4428

Antineoplaston

Dr. Stanislaw Burzynski of Houston, Texas has discovered a cancer therapy called antineoplaston. The antineoplastons interrupt the function of oncogenes, which stimulate the growths of tumors and stimulate the tumor suppressor genes. They do not kill cells, but *normalize cell growth.*

The antineoplastons appear to be particularly effective in treatment of brain tumors, which are not cured by conventional chemotherapy. It is also helpful in other tumors. The therapy is quite safe.

A Japanese university president suffering from cancer of the colon that had spread to the liver came to Houston for treatment. He is now well. *Chemotherapy has been unable to cure any cancers that have spread into the liver.*

A patient of Dr. Julian Whitaker developed low grade non - Hodgekin's lymphoma in 1991, for which there was no curative therapy. She was started on antineoplaston therapy and her tumors began to shrink in three weeks and complete remission was present within twelve weeks. She remains well ten years later.

Noni

Noni is a Polynesian fruit that has wonderful healing attributes. At least two persons with cancer started taking Noni and recovered. One of these persons had been given only two weeks to live when Noni was started. The second patient had breast cancer and refused to have surgery. This is not a guaranteed cure, of course, but these and other cases suggest it might be worthwhile to try.

NONI comes in 32 ounce bottles and I would suggest taking 2 ounces twice daily until you are certain you are getting better. Then the dose could be decreased to one or two ounces twice daily.

Noni is available in health food stores and through *Natural Health Team*. There are no side effects.

The Abortion Breast Cancer Cover-Up

More than 30 studies have confirmed a relationship between having an abortion and the subsequent development of breast cancer.

Since 1960 there has been a surge in the number of women developing breast cancer in the USA. Currently every woman in this nation has between a 10 and 12% chance of developing breast cancer.

In November 1994, a National Cancer Institute (NCI) study done at the Hutchinson Cancer Research Center in Seattle, Wash. showed a clear link between abortion and the development of breast cancer.

Dr. Joel Brind, Professor of Biology and Endocrinology at Baruch College of the City College of New York has been crusading to get the information that abortion is a major factor in the causation of breast cancer to the public. Not one magazine or newspaper was willing to print his findings. His research was finally reported in Lancet, a fine English medical journal.

When you enter a Planned Parenthood Clinic to have an abortion do they tell you that this procedure increases your chance of breast cancer by 50%? If a woman has an abortion at anytime, her chance of developing breast cancer goes up by at least 50%.

The NCI research disclosed that if the abortion was performed before age 18, the risk was increased by 150%. If the woman was over 30 and had a family history of mother, sister, grandmother, or aunt with breast cancer the risk went up by 270%. *The most ominous finding was that every woman who had an abortion before age 18 and had a family history of breast cancer developed breast cancer by the age of 45.* There were only 12 women in this study who fit this category, but they all developed breast cancer. (Source: November 1994 National Cancer Institute report of a study performed at the Fred Hutchinson Cancer Research Center, Seattle, Washington).

A Howard University study in December 1993 confirmed the NCI findings but had a longer follow up. By the time the women who had an abortion reached the age of 50 the chance of breast cancer had increased by 370%.

The story for multiple abortions is even worse. The more abortions a woman has the greater the risk of breast cancer. A study from France showed that a woman with a family history of breast cancer who had 2 or more abortions increased her risk of breast cancer 6 fold.

In Lithuania it is common for women to have had 5 abortions by the time they reach 25. *They are experiencing an explosive increase in breast cancer in young women.*

Many women believe that there is nothing wrong with having an abortion. Proverbs 14:12 states" There is a way that seems right unto man, but the end thereof is death." *Abortion not only kills the child it jeopardizes the life of the mother.*

Why does abortion increase the chance of breast cancer?

Dr. Brind believes that abortion leaves the breast cells in a permanent suspended state where they are neither dormant nor mature and that these cells are susceptible to undergo malignant change.

Breast Care

Carcinogenic agents are often found in breast tissue and fluid discharged from the nipple. These fluids show DDT, PCB's, dioxins, and heavy metals in breast milk. These carcinogenic materials contribute to breast cancer *especially if they remain static.*

During nipple stimulation and orgasm in nursing mothers, post reproductive, premenopausal or postmenopausal women, oxytocin is produced and this helps clear the breast of trapped secretions. This affords a good explanation for why the incidence of breast cancer is lower among sexually active women than non-sexually active women of the same age.

Dr. Timothy Murrell of the University of Adelaide has observed that women frequently overlook nipple care and present themselves with atrophic, small, flat and scaly nipples. This neglect leads to obstruction of glands. These changes can be reversed within four menstrual cycles by careful regular nipple stimulation.

Dr. Murrell also thinks that tight compressive clothing may inhibit circulation in the breast. This could explain the incidence of breast cancer being higher in cold climates than in warm. Vitamin D lack in cold climates is also a possible explanation.

Organochlorines And Breast Cancer

To the hazards which clearly contribute towards breast cancer, hormones (estrogen), high- fat diet, abortion and family history there is one more problem. That is *organochlorines*.

There are more than 10,000 different organochlorines, including chlordane, DDT, dioxin, vinyl chloride, atrazine, and CFCs. Studies routinely show that women with breast cancer have high tissue levels of organochlorines . *Farmers and chemical workers who are exposed to organochlorines have high levels of breast cancer.* Organochlorines take time to do their damage, rather than cause acute toxic problems. They accumulate in fatty tissue such as breast. Excretion is very slow.

How To Minimize Your Exposure

Eat only organic produce. Wash produce with mild soap and water.

Use nontoxic or natural pesticides. Always wear gloves when using a pesticide to prevent skin absorption.

Be sure your drinking water has no organochlorines. This is best accomplished with filtered water.

General Measures To Assist Recovery From Cancer

Everything that can improve an individual's *general health* should be done. We know that alcohol and smoking damage the bone marrow. If you are going to continue smoking 2 packs of cigarettes and drinking a fifth of whiskey daily, *even flax oil and cottage cheese may not be able to help.* Eat the best possible foods with plenty of organic vegetables and fruit. Strongly consider juicing fruit and vegetables, as this insures the full benefit of the nutrients without any possible loss of value from cooking. The same benefit occurs with eating raw food and vegetables.

If you fear cancer, please read Dr. William Fischer's book *How To Fight Cancer And Win.* This is a scholarly, scientific book which documents several other *natural* treatments (those of Dr. Max Gerson, Dr. Hans Nieper, Dr. Josef Issels, William Kelly, Dr. Cornelius Moerman, Gaston Naessens) that have reportedly worked in some cases. This book is available from Agora Health Books of Baltimore, Md.

There is no guaranteed cure for cancer. However, numerous natural treatments have shown very promising results in some people. Considering the alternatives, they are certainly worth exploring if you, a family member or friends have cancer.

Chapter 15

The Truth About Sunlight

John Ott has done monumental work in the field of photobiology. This work has proven that the full spectrum of visible light (and some of the invisible) is absolutely essential for good health. Ott has shown that light is just as important a photosynthesing mechanism in animals as it is in plants; only the mechanism is different.

In the June 1990 issue of The Reader's Digest Dr. David Ruben wrote an article about ultraviolet light blaming 600,000 cases of skin cancer annually on this form of light. He goes on to say that exposing their bodies to the sunlight is one of the riskiest things Americans can do.

Blaming the ultraviolet light from the sun for skin cancer appears to be incorrect. The skin cancer problem is not caused by ultraviolet light. In Australia skin cancer is two times more common in persons eating margarine instead of butter. Butter has an ingredient that appears to prevent the development of skin cancer. *The skin cancer seen in Australia occurs more in office workers than those employed outdoors.*

Dr. Wayne London, a medical researcher at Dartmouth Medical School, has written Health Benefits of Full Spectrum Light and Light and the Immune System which summarize his views. His conclusions are:

Full spectrum light benefits rheumatoid arthritis and multiple sclerosis;

Phototherapy, which uses ultraviolet light (UV), is effective treatment for psoriasis;

Two types of cancer (breast and colon) have been associated with either a lack of light or blocking of full spectrum light;

Patients with candida(yeast) respond to supplemental full spectrum light. They also experience an increase in lymphocytes in the peripheral blood.

John Ott states that we need more ultraviolet light than we obtain from artificial light through windows. Ultraviolet light of the short wave length, germicidal ultraviolet, is mostly filtered out by the earth's atmosphere. *This fear of getting too much ultraviolet light is creating a deficiency of an essential life supporting energy.*

Ott further relates that there is probably a relationship between chronic diseases and lack of sunlight." My studies have shown that light is a nutrient, similar to all the other nutrients we take in through food and that we need the full spectrum range of natural sunlight". If human skin is not exposed to solar radiation (direct or scattered) for long periods of time, disturbances will occur in the physiological equilibrium of the human system. The result will be disorders of the nervous system, vitamin D deficiency, weakening of the body's defenses, and an aggravation of chronic diseases".

He calls this state *malillumination* (lack of necessary sunlight). This develops when wavelengths are missing in various types of artificial light or are filtered from natural light passing through window glass, windshields, tinted eyeglasses, smog, and sun tan lotions. The minerals and chemicals in the individual cells of our bodies that would normally be metabolized by the missing wavelengths *remain in the equivalent of darkness.*

In other words energy cannot be extracted from food materials if the proper wavelengths are not obtained to help break them down chemically.

Dr. Ott has called the attention of the medical profession to the dangers of using tinted eyeglasses. He has perfected gray-tinted lenses that will allow the passage of all wavelengths of light. The majority of sunglasses available today do not permit full transmission of light and are *clearly detrimental to the health of the wearer.*

We are all exposed to all the rays of the energy spectrum, including cosmic, x-ray, visible light, infrared, and radio. It would be simplistic to think these ubiquitous rays are not related to our vital life processes both in positive and negative ways.

Dr. Ott compares the skin to solar cells used by satellites to obtain energy from the sun. The layering of the skin is similar to the layering of the different elements that are used to make capacitors, condensers, transistors, and flashlight batteries. The langerhans cells are located between basal cells and prickel cells. They have dendrites which give them the potential to transmit and are our bodies' biologic solar energy cells. We, just like a pot of geraniums, need direct sunlight for good health.

An interesting and controversial study was carried out in a Sarasota, Florida grade school at Ott's suggestion. Two windowless classrooms were equipped with Ott's radiation shielded full-spectrum fluorescent lights. Two identical classrooms were equipped with standard cool white fluorescent lights to be used as controls. Cameras equipped to do time lapse photography were placed in all four classrooms to permit monitoring of all children's behavior.

The cameras recording the activity of the children exposed to full spectrum light recorded a marked decrease in hyperactivity among the children, with a definite calming effect and an increase in their attention span compared to those in cool white non- full- spectrum light. In particular, several extremely hyperactive children with "confirmed learning disabilities" calmed down and *rapidly reversed their learning disabilities under full spectrum light.*

One little boy, who stood out in the earlier films because he was always in motion and was inattentive, had changed to a quieter child able to sit still and concentrate on classroom routine. His teacher related that he was capable of doing independent study now and that *he had even learned to read during this short observation period.*

The children in the "normal" classroom were photographed fidgeting to an extreme degree, leaping from their seats, flailing their arms, and paying little attention to their teachers.

The overall academic achievement level of those exposed to full spectrum light was superior to those under the deficient lights, and, perhaps the most incredible finding of all, dentists confirmed that the children in full spectrum light had one third fewer cavities. *Dr. Ott offered to donate the lights for the continued health of the children but the offer was refused.*

Dr. Ott did another study with cancer patients, *which showed clear prolongation of life.* He advised 15 cancer patients to spend as much time as possible in sunlight and to avoid artificial light sources including television. 14 of the 15 showed no progression of their tumors and several actually showed improvement. The one person who failed to improve had misunderstood the directions and *continued to wear sunglasses.*

In another study the heart cells of chicks, when subjected to red light, weakened and ultimately ruptured. This raised the question could there be a connection between the high red content of ordinary incandescent lights and the high frequency of coronary disorders. No one followed up on this information.

In a study of fish breeding, fish hatched under pink light were almost all females. Rats born under full spectrum ultraviolet light had a high survival rate, whereas, those under pink fluorescent light had only 61% survivors. Mice left under a pink fluorescent light for 6 months developed rotting of their tails, which fell off.

There is danger from the ends of fluorescent tubes and television sets caused by x-radiation. Plants placed near the ends of fluorescent tubes will not grow.

The hyperactive reaction to radiation from unshielded fluorescent tubes or television may correlate with the hyperactive symptoms and severe learning disorders triggered by artificial food flavors and colorings. Dr. Ben Feingold of the Kaiser Permanente Foundation Hospital in San Francisco found that a diet eliminating all foods containing artificial flavors and colors brought about dramatic improvement in 15 of 25 hyperactive children. *Any infraction of the diet led to hyperactive behavior within a few hours.*

In a study in a Adjustive Education Center for hyperactive children in Sarasota Dr. Ott was able to get the home TV sets which had excessive radiation either repaired or discarded. Additionally, all TV sets that backed up against a wall where someone was working or sleeping were moved. Parents enforced the number of hours TV could be watched and *children were encouraged to sit far away from the TV set.* The principal noted that improved behavior was found in *all* children in homes where defective radiation of TV sets led to repair or discarding. One of the children who had been sleeping on the other side of a wall where the TV was giving off .3 milliroentgens of radiation per hour improved so markedly *she was returned to a normal school.*

Young rats were placed close to a color TV set whose picture tube was covered with black photographic paper. These rats became very stimulated then lethargic. *They all died in 10 to 12 days.*

Conventional medical authorities claim ultraviolet light from sunlight causes cataracts. The cataracts are actually caused by the *infrared part of the spectrum.* Glass blowers are constantly looking into a furnace that emits infrared light not ultraviolet light. They get a special cataract called "glass blower's cataract".

Most people are constantly irradiated by *infrared* from incandescent light bulbs, which peak at the infrared portion of the spectrum. In Australia and other areas of very high light intensity *skin cancer is more common in office workers than those who work in sunlight.*

Ultraviolet deprivation may be responsible for the dramatic increase in cancer seen in certain parts of Africa. Albert Schweitzer noted that when he arrived in Africa the natives did not wear sunglasses and that he rarely saw cancer. Later natives could be seen pulling their canoes down the river wearing sunglasses and not much else. The failure to receive ultraviolet through their eyes because of sunglasses made them vulnerable to ultraviolet light deficiency as black skinned persons do not absorb much ultraviolet through their skin.

This ill advised fear of ultraviolet light has made employees at the Bureau of Radiologic Health of the U.S. Food and Drug Administration very vulnerable to bad health! All fluorescent tubes in their labs and offices have been outfitted with a special ultraviolet filtering sleeve of plastic as well as a plastic diffuser for ultraviolet in every fluorescent fixture. This confirms the Douglass Rule of Inverse Government Action (DRIGA). The more the government tries to solve a problem, the worse the problem gets.

Niles, Illinois had a school with a very high rate of leukemia. Ott visited the school and discovered that the curtains filtering the outside light caused a greenish glow. The fluorescent lights in the room were emitting a strong orange pink part of the spectrum. After removal of the drapes so sunlight entered the room and placing full spectrum fluorescent lights *no new cases of leukemia were seen.*

Ott is convinced that the inability of women to become pregnant is related to use of tinted sunglasses. *He advised 6 women to throw away their sunglasses and they all became pregnant.* Estrogen, an essential hormone for conception, has a sharp peak in absorption of ultraviolet light at 280 nanometers. This frequency of light is usually filtered out by sunglasses and this causes failure of proper activation of estrogen with inability to conceive.

Seasonal Affective Disorders (SAD)

John Ott's work Seasonal Affective Disorders has become a fairly common well accepted syndrome which occurs in fall and winter due to light deficiency. Patients with this disorder develop fatigue; sadness, excessive sleeping, overeating, carbohydrate craving and weight gain during the short days of winter. These changes can be reversed by extending the light period using 5 to 6 hours of bright, 2500 lux, full spectrum light either in the morning and evening hours or evening hours alone. The anti-depressive effects of this treatment take two to four days to appear, and relapse in the same number of days occurs if treatment is stopped. These behavioral improvements are believed to be caused by decreased secretion of melatonin from the pineal gland in a light enhanced environment.

Four percent of persons living in middle latitudes have the SAD disorder. There is a summer version of the problem called Summer SAD. This condition occurs in July and August and is characterized by agitation, insomnia and weight loss. Both types of SAD are most common in women aged 21 to 40. Winter SAD affects only 1.4% of persons in Florida whereas in New Hampshire, the incidence approaches 10%. Alaska also manifests a 10% incidence of winter SAD.

Patients with SAD show a different pattern of conception. The usual peak period for conception is in December but patients with SAD have a peak period for conception in late summer. Dr. Douglass feels that the SAD syndrome is probably related to ultraviolet lack and could be helped by photo-oxidation.

If you know a person with SAD have them contact International Bio-oxidation Medicine Foundation(IBOM) at 405-5575127. Encourage them to throw away their sunglasses and get full spectrum lighting at home and work.

These lights can be ordered by writing Health Lighting Inc., P.O. Box 728, Dahlonega, Ga.30533-0728 or calling 800-557 5127.

In tropical nations, where exposure to sunlight is normal, the incidence of osteoporosis, hip and spinal fracture, cataracts, and colon and breast cancer is less common. The lack of sunlight seen in cold climates in winter causes a failure of adequate vitamin D production which damages the immune system and may lead to more cancer than is seen in warm climates where vitamin D levels tend to be higher.

In the American Journal of Clinical Nutrition, Dr. Reinhold Veith of the University of Toronto proposed that the daily intake of vitamin D should be increased to 800 to 1000 units daily. Because we are getting less vitamin D from our food than previously and because many individuals are covered with sunscreens which block the production of Vitamin D this seems like a good idea particularly in northern climates.

Chapter 16

Skin Diseases

As mentioned above, there is a strong suspicion that widespread use of sunscreens may actually be *increasing* the number of cases of skin cancer. Sunscreens prevent the body from producing melanin, which is capable of absorbing the various frequencies of ultraviolet light. Without the melanin deposit the skin continues to be injured by ultraviolet light.

The problem of rising numbers of cases of skin cancer may also be related to worldwide changes in dietary fat intake. Dangerous transfats from synthetic oils and margarines have replaced butter, lard, coconut oil, olive oil and flax oil in our diet.

Researchers in Australia studied patients who had contracted melanoma and compared these individuals with a test control group. Those persons who had melanoma *consumed twice the quantity of margarine as persons without melanoma.* These investigators suggested substituting butter for margarine. They also recommended adding Omega 3 fatty acids to the diet (salmon, trout, tuna, mackerel, and sardines.) along with flax oil or seeds, walnuts, and pumpkin seeds.

The current popular idea of what causes skin cancer blames the disease on loss of ozone and more vacation time spent in the sunlight.

However, that's not entirely true. Look at the following: fifteen years ago skin cancer was not a serious problem in Mexico. Instead of afflicting a few elderly persons, there are now eight and a half million persons with skin cancer in Mexico.

What caused this?

The reason: there was a fundamental change in the way Mexicans eat. Instead of using lard to cook, margarine, hydrogenated shortening and vegetable oils are used. Clever advertising has convinced the populace that these hydrogenated fats are healthier. *Not so.*

The second problem produced by these dietary changes is a skyrocketing incidence of heart and artery problems. As mentioned earlier, *hydrogenated fats are an artificial product that are hard for the body to eliminate.* These artificial, abnormal fats raise the level of LDL (bad) cholesterol and decrease the level of HDL (good) cholesterol. This change results in arteriosclerosis and heart attacks. When Mexicans return to lard or butter for cooking and stop using margarine, artificial shortenings and salad oil they may see their heart disease and skin cancer rates recede.

Neem

Neem is an Indian product that you are likely to hear much more about in the future. The neem tree is similar to mahogany and grows well in poor soil. Grinding the seeds and leaves creates a *natural pesticide* harmless to humans. Scrubbing the teeth with a frayed twig of this tree keeps teeth very healthy.

Neem works well to eliminate viral, bacterial and fungal infections. I have applied neem to fungal infections and found the itching and redness to be better within 48 hours. Crude extracts of neem make an excellent insect repellant.

The neem oil can be purchased from Ayurvedic Institute 505-291 9698

Skin Answer

A glycoalkaloid derived from the "devil's apple" plant from Australia has been modified in the USA into a product that reportedly dissolves basal cell and squamous cell cancers of the skin in three to four weeks. This product takes advantage of the *increased permeability* of skin cancer cells to a glycoalkaloid, when compared to normal skin.

The malignant cell is injured by the glycoalkaloid enzymes and explodes. The cancer cell is then replaced by healthy normal cells. This should be applied twice daily. An interesting facet of this therapy is that pre-cancerous skin lesions called actinic keratosis also disappear with Skin Answer. This product can be obtained from CompassioNet: 800-510 2010

Vitiligo

Vitiligo is a skin disorder, manifested by de-pigmented areas of skin. It is often slowly progressive and has been hard to treat. The disease has been regarded as one of the autoimmune disorders, in which the body appears to 'attack" it's own cells. There is sometimes association with other autoimmune diseases (diabetes mellitus, pernicious anemia, Addison's Disease, thyroiditis and hyperthyroidism).

Researchers in Sweden have discovered that high doses of B 12 and folic acid can improve vitiligo.

Psoriasis

My first suggestion for psoriasis would be to try thymic extract. (See Chapter 3 Immune Illness). Use of thymic extract had arrested 12 cases of psoriasis. (Health Sciences Institute Member Alert March 1998)

The second suggestion is an extract of the Oregon Grape (mahonia aquifolium, or MA). This was given to 433 patients with psoriasis in Germany in 1995. Over 12 weeks the dermatologists reported that symptoms improved or completely disappeared in 81% of cases.

In one case, Paula had suffered from psoriasis for 60 years. Within one month of MA, her psoriasis was gone. There is an MA shampoo, which works well for the common scalp lesions. This product can be obtained from Great Britain.

Borage Oil

Borage oil is made from the seeds of borage, a wildflower known as starflower. Borage oil is a rich source of the essential fatty acid gamma linolenic acid (GLA). Humans are able to make adequate amounts of GLA from linoleic acid, a fatty acid found in all edible vegetable oils. This GLA is converted into Prostaglandin 1 (PG 1) an important compound, which has an effective anti-inflammatory action and also regulates water loss from the skin and protects the skin from injury.

Persons with atopic dermatitis, eczema and psoriasis often show high levels of linoleic acid but low levels of GLA, suggesting failure to convert linoleic acid from the diet into GLA. The low levels of PG 1 may be the cause for dry skin and water loss from the skin seen in these three conditions

The use of borage oil permits the body to directly receive GLA. Oral ingestion of borage oil has been shown to increase PG 1 levels in the skin and stop inflammation. Borage oil is commonly found in health food stores.

Trienelle Daily Renewal Cream (TDRC)

This cream is reported to promptly restore a more normal healthy appearance to aging skin. Two of the key ingredients in this substance are natural tocotrienols extracted from Malaysian palm kernels and Japanese rice bran oil. *Tocotrienals are an unusual form of Vitamin E* that has profound skin protective properties.

The Tocular Skin Nutrition Complex combines the tocotrienols with other enzymatic antioxidants and cofactors delivered by liposomes. After smoothing on the skin, the liposome penetrates deeply into the skin and slowly releases antioxidants at a steady rate.

Aging skin loses firmness and elasticity. The proper care of the skin depends on the *underlying* collagen tissue. As the collagen-supporting network weakens with aging, the skin becomes slack with folding, lines, and the appearance of wrinkles.

Ultraviolet light exposure increases the production of collagenase, which breaks down the collagen fibers permitting wrinkles to appear. Additionally, ultraviolet light slows the production of new collagen.

Researchers in France have found a special molecule containing the amino acids lysine, threonine and serine that resemble a small piece of collagen. This molecule is able to replenish the collagen matrix, which helps restore the tautness and elasticity of the skin. This molecule contributes to creating firmer young appearing skin.

The TDRC also contains colostrum from New Zealand, extracts of reishi and other Japanese mushrooms, and alpha hydroxy acids (AHA). The AHA appears to smooth out wrinkles and lines.

TDRC has a skin protection factor of 15. Some of the other nutrients in TDRC include applephenone (an antioxidant from green apples), melatonin (an anti-aging antioxidant), mixed carotenoids, phytosterols (which are natural plant lipids that nurture and enhance skin luster), and co-enzyme Q10 a powerful antioxidant.

TDRC appears to be a valuable product capable of restoring healthier skin. A one or two month trial could prove rewarding.

This can be obtained from Aspen Benefits Group, 877-432 7891.

Baldness

Scottish researchers have discovered that nightly massage of the scalp with the essential oils, thyme, rosemary, lavender, and cedar wood may bring about hair growth in cases of alopecia areata. Alopecia areata is a skin disorder, which causes bald patches to appear in the scalp, eyebrows, beard, and other hairy areas. Forty four per cent of the patients taking the essential oils showed improvement, when compared to a control group.

Dr. Victor Marcial-Vega, who has wide experience with essential oils in his practice at the Health Horizons Clinic in Coral Gables, Florida says, "all these essential oils are highly stimulating to the circulation, which is helpful for stimulating hair growth. In addition, each has specific cleansing properties. The cedar wood and rosemary are both antibacterial and thyme is a powerful antifungal agent. Lavender is known to enhance skin and wound healing, as well as being a stress reducer".

Dr. Marcial-Vega explains that this blend appears to cleanse the scalp of any bacterial or fungal organisms that may effect the health of the skin and interfere with hair growth and brings additional blood and nutrients to the scalp. Dr. Marcial-Vega relates "So far, we are seeing good results, not only for alopecia areata, but also for age related hair thinning, stress related hair loss, and the hair loss induced by chemotherapy drugs. The results with male pattern hair loss are comparable to Rogaine".

Essential oils are concentrated essences of medicinal plants. They can be absorbed into the body by ingestion, rubbing on the skin, or inhaled as a vapor. These essential oils contain tiny molecules of pharmacologically active substances that affect various body systems, including the immune system and the central nervous system. The molecules are easily absorbed through the skin, digestive tract, or mucous membranes of the nose, throat, and lungs.

Many essential oils are highly antiseptic, exhibiting anti- viral, anti-bacterial, and anti- fungal properties. Others are capable of affecting brain wave patterns, leading to stimulation or sedation.

Often an essential oil will exhibit properties similar to the herb it was made from, but is far more potent. For example, a tea made from anise seed is a good digestive aid, relieving indigestion and flatulence, while a single drop of anise seed oil can relieve gastrointestinal cramps.

To use for baldness, place one drop of essential oil product on each finger of one hand. The fingers are rubbed together to warm the oil and then the scalp is massaged for 2 to 5 minutes nightly at bedtime. Persons who have redness, irritation or itching of the scalp should specify that they wish to use Hair Blend containing thyme, which clears infections.

Hair Blend Oil can be obtained from Health Horizons 305 442-1233 or 1800 771-0255 or from our *Natural Health Team*.

Chapter 17

Gastrointestinal Diseases

The bacteria in our intestinal tract are very important to good health. They:

- Improve the function of the whole gastrointestinal tract

- Protect our body against pathogenic bacteria entering the gastrointestinal tract

- Produce needed vitamins and hormones

- Maintain chemical balance of the gastrointestinal tract

There are more than 400 species of bacteria in our gut and their total weight varies from 2 pounds to 4 pounds. In the large bowel, there may be as many as one trillion bacteria per ml. Probiotic substances are the healthy bacteria found in yogurt, kefir, sour milk, cheese and acidophilus milk etc., which contribute to the health and balance of the gastrointestinal tract.

Normally the ph of the gastrointestinal tract is acidic 5.0 to 6.9. When the ph becomes alkaline (above 7), problems may appear including the passage of food particles into the blood (leaky gut syndrome) which may cause allergy to these foreign particles.

The using of pesticides for farming along with fertilizers, destroyed much of the soil based bacteria usually residing in the gastrointestinal tract. Sterilizing water with chlorine further reduced beneficial bacteria in the intestinal tract.

As this sterilization of soil and water proceeded, there was a corresponding decrease in the beneficial bacteria found in our bodies. Normally the balance is 85% good and 15% bad. *This ratio is now reversed for most Americans.* This contributes to the rising problem of chronic degenerative illnesses and gastrointestinal symptoms.

Two common good bacteria in our gut are lactobacilli and disporidium. These good bacteria do several valuable things:

- Stimulate the immunologic function of the spleen

- Create a protective barrier against harmful organisms by coating the intestinal lining.

- Compete with harmful organisms for nutrients thus keeping their population down.

- Produce beneficial natural antibiotic substances such as acidophillin, bifidin, and hydrogen peroxide.

- Aid in the fermentation of soluble fiber, which yields short chain fatty acids *that supply between 5 and 10% of human energy needs.*

- Increase the bio-availability of calcium

The delicate balance of these helpful bacteria can be disturbed by a diet that is too high in sugar or one that is too low in natural fermented milk products (yogurt, cottage cheese, whey, buttermilk, sauerkraut).

Excessive consumption of alcohol and the drinking of fluoridated or chlorinated water can also disturb the balance of these needed bacteria.

Radiation therapy and the use of non-steroidal anti-inflammatory drugs like motrin, advil, nuprin, rufin, medipren, etc. also injure these bacteria.

The most serious damage occurs after taking a course of antibiotics. This kills nearly all the good bacteria. This enables the surviving bacteria, which are mostly bad, to multiply and become the predominant organism. This is the reason doctors often tell patients, as I did, "*I don't want to put you on an antibiotic because I am sure your infection is viral. The antibiotic will not help the virus, but it may leave you with diarrhea, vomiting and or a yeast infection.* "

Supplementing your diet with yogurt, cottage cheese, sauerkraut or replenishing the gastrointestinal bacteria with Culturelle can often help these problems.

Culturelle was discovered in 1985. This is lactobacillus G.G., which can treat candidiasis, protect against food borne aflatoxins, treat all forms of diarrhea and help produce immune chemicals that may help prevent cancer. When refrigerated for as long as 6 months, Culturelle can deliver 20 billion live bacteria per capsule. The dose is one capsule daily. This product can be obtained from Vitamin Research Products 800-877-2447

Soil Based Organisms (SBO)

This natural substance is fascinating to me. There are indications that it has beneficial effects on the immune system.

If anyone had asked me if I thought taking soil based organisms could cure someone of intractable petit mal epilepsy, my answer would have been, of course not. There is no way I would believe that taking a natural bacteria by mouth could break up an abnormal electrical discharge from the brain, which is what epilepsy is. Yet, a 14-year-old boy ceased having petit mal epilepsy after starting SBO.

What Are Soil Based Organisms?

These are tiny microbes that live in the soil. They release powerful enzymes that sterilize the soil of putrefying bacteria, thus preparing the soil to support new plant growth. Without SBO, the soil would be overrun with yeasts, molds, fungi, candida and other harmful organisms that antagonize plant growth and reproduction. SBO also produce and release nutrients and growth hormones that get absorbed through the roots of the plants and help stimulate reproduction by the plants.

As the SBO grow, partly because of their own growth hormone stimulating production there is a geometric increase in the hormones in the area, which accelerates seed development and plant growth.

In the 1800's, people ate SBO from raw fruit and vegetables with favorable consequences. Modern technology with pesticides, fungicides, and heat based food processing kill most of the SBO.

There is speculation that the declining intake of SBO is one reason that Americans have more bowel and digestive disorders than people in countries where this high tech farming and food processing have not yet appeared.

SBO were discovered by a scientist as a large clump above the surface of the ground. These bacteria were found to be safe for fingerling fish and they actually stimulated growth of these fish. Further research by Peter Smith enabled the bacteria to be screened for superior qualities and to also have the capability to produce specific and startling healing and immune stimulating effects.

SBO are found in a product called Earth Flora and is a gray black powder with micronutrients and phytoplankton which act as a substrate for the live SBO. The SBO are dormant until introduced into water or juice. *There is a shelf life of 5 years at room temperature and longer if refrigerated. No toxic side effects have been uncovered after 12 years of use.*

Persons using this substance consistently claim to have virtual immunity to colds and flu, stronger digestive capability, elimination of constipation and other chronic gastrointestinal symptoms, increased metabolism, increased energy, increased strength, quick healing of wounds and increased mental clarity.

When taken by mouth the SBO attach to the wall of the whole digestive tract. The bacteria grow and multiply into large colonies wherever they attach. They greatly increase the body's ability to absorb and utilize crucial nutrients, while simultaneously ridding the intestinal tract of putrefying and disease- causing organisms.

The five main functions of SBO:

- They eliminate putrified material, where harmful bacteria live. They actually devour this material off the wall of the colon so it is easily eliminated.

- The SBO's break down hydrocarbons into small particles that are easily absorbed, which have a dramatic beneficial effect on overall nutrition. Constipation often disappears overnight.

- These SBO's produce specific proteins which act as antigens. This stimulates the immune system to produce far beyond the usual quantity of specific protein. This amplifies the immune systems ability to ward off disease. Also the immune system has a greatly enhanced ability to combat any illness in that person.

- All pathogenic molds, yeast, fungi, viruses, and harmful organisms, which might cause illness or a chronic degenerative disease are ingested and disappear. This permits the harassed and overworked immune system to rest and get restored.

- The SBO's work to metabolize proteins for the cells while simultaneously ridding the cells of toxic wastes, thus boosting health of the cell.

New Immune Discoveries About SBO

Stimulation of Body's Natural Alpha Interferon Production

Alpha interferon is a key regulator of the body's immune responses. The use of recombinant technology to create alpha interferon has not been very successful because it is very expensive to manufacture and the end product is a single subspecies of alpha interferon. (There are known to be *20* subspecies of alpha interferon.) This necessitates huge doses, which have a very low effect on the immune stimulation response and are very toxic. *Natural* alpha interferon produced by the human body exerts a very powerful immune response involving all 20 subspecies.

The reason the body makes so many different subspecies of alpha interferon is that different subspecies are needed to combat different viruses and other antigens. *No one species can protect against the wide variety of harmful invaders that attack the body. Laboratory studies have shown that SBO stimulates at least 16 of the 20 subspecies.* This ability to stimulate a wide spectrum of *the body's own* alpha interferon may be the reason why SBO appears to benefit such a wide variety of chronic degenerative problems, such as chronic fatigue syndrome, hepatitis B and C, influenza, and others.

In summary, it appears that SBO's ability to stimulate the majority of the human subspecies of alpha interferon leads to greatly increased T lymphocyte production and the anti-viral capability of the immune system is augmented, as a direct effect of the increased production of alpha interferon. This is all a very beneficial effect and protection for the body.

Stimulation Of B Lymphocytes And Related Antibody Production

Once established in the gastrointestinal tract, the SBO's produce a protein mass regarded by the body as a foreign substance. This generates the *production of huge quantities of B lymphocytes, which make huge quantities of antibody.*

This antibody is unique in that it is non-directed, i.e. it has not been programmed to attack a specific infection or pathogenic agent. These antibodies are kept in reserve for the body to use whenever needed for whatever needed.

When an infection appears, the immune system is able to immediately imprint precisely the awaiting reservoir antibody with information to attack the invader. This leads to rapid recovery.

This means that the individual with this reservoir of antibody has a greatly enhanced immune system compared to persons not taking SBO. These SBO's should give the individual using them greater protection from infection than was previously possible. There are no known side effects and unlikely to be, since they are a natural substance.

Crucial Lactoferrin Supplementation To The Body

Dr. Rothschild discovered that the SBO's also produced lactoferrin in humans as a byproduct of their metabolism. Lactoferrin is a vital element to humans as it retrieves iron from our ingested food and then delivers the iron to sites where the body needs iron.

Frequently, lactoferrin levels in the body are not high and those persons may have trouble assimilating iron. Iron deficiency anemia is usually caused by internal bleeding from the gastrointestinal tract, but can follow chronic bleeding from any site. At times, an anemia resembling blood loss fails to improve with iron therapy. This has been termed the *Anemia of Chronic Illness.*

In retrospect, these persons may have inadequate lactoferrin levels to absorb iron properly. Dr. Rothschild states that less than 50% of the persons with iron deficiency symptoms suffer from inadequate iron in their diet. They're taking iron in, but it's not clearing up the iron deficiency. When these persons take supplemental iron, the extra iron does not end up in red blood cells, but there is a *surplus* of iron in the body.

This is a bonanza for the harmful yeasts, bacteria, viruses and parasites, which all have a continuous need for iron and tend to thrive in an iron rich environment. However, when iron is carried through the body by lactoferrin, 95% is assimilated and the tight bond to lactoferrin prevents use by viruses, bacteria, yeasts, and parasites. In this manner, lactoferrin acts as a defense against invading pathogens. In effect it starves pathogens of a vitally needed material (iron).

Stimulates Cellular Repair

The SBO's produce much DNA and RNA, which is coded to activate self repair in certain human cells. This is believed to explain why patients with severe burns, skin ulcers, non- healing surgical incisions and infected wounds appear to heal faster with SBO.

Super Oxide Desmutase

Super oxide desmutase (SOD) is a byproduct of SBO metabolism in humans. SOD is a powerful enzyme and cellular antioxidant that acts as a super scavenger of dangerous free radicals throughout the body. Very few foods contain SOD, so many persons are lacking this substance.

Studies at Johns Hopkins University have shown that SOD can diminish heart damage after a heart attack. This may be because the enzymatic activity of SOD permits improved energy production within cells, helping them nourish and repair themselves in a more efficient manner.

Correct Deficient Nutrient Absorption

This quality of SBO enables an individual to obtain all needed items from the diet. Dr.Rothschild claims that the mineral deficit is more indicative of *faulty absorption* than of lack of needed nutrients in the diet. The micronutrients of SBO are believed to be easy to assimilate and they teach the body how to assimilate the higher nutrient levels provided by the diet. Some of these micronutrients are actually byproducts of metabolism of SBO's.

Other micronutrients are contained within the SBO organism and become available to the human for absorption when the SBO dies. Among these 71 nutrients are chlorophyll, phytocyanin, amino acids, vitamins including B 12, minerals, SOD, bromelain, nucleic acids proteins, beta carotene, and gamma linoleic acid, an essential fatty acid. The dosages of these micronutrients are so tiny they are rapidly and easily absorbed. They then act as biologic response modifiers, which make it easier for the same nutrient to be absorbed in a larger dosage.

What Has SBO Done In Patients?

I have already mentioned the fascinating recovery of the young man from petit mal epilepsy. A second case is of considerable interest: The patient was a man with a serious urinary tract obstruction from an enlarged prostate. He was scheduled for prostate surgery and received SBO for several weeks prior to the surgery, to improve his healing after the surgery. When the time for the operation arrived *it was discovered that his prostate gland had returned to normal size and the surgery was cancelled.* To me, this is equally as mysterious as the cessation of petit mal epilepsy after SBO.

A third case which intrigued me was an Englishwoman who received 11 ten day courses of antibiotics. Following the antibiotic treatments, she became profoundly intolerant of all food and had to survive on a liquid diet of predigested drinks for three months. Her weight fell by 28 pounds.

She visited 14 alternative care practitioners and many physicians. Her stool cultures showed *no beneficial bacteria.* Taking acidophilus and bifidus led to no improvement. In the book *Beyond Probiotics* by Ann Gittleman she read about SBO and began this therapy. Initially, she took one capsule weekly. This was increased by one capsule each week until she took 15 each day. There were many ups and downs in her course, but she gradually got better. She regained the lost weight and now *is eating food she could never tolerate.*

There have been reports of remissions of cancer, Parkinson's disease, glaucoma, nervous disorders and high cholesterol after use of SBO. The return of a prostate gland to normal size after several weeks of SBO is surprising.

There is clear evidence that SBO strengthens our immune system as well as benefiting gastrointestinal problems..

Who Should Consider A Trial Of SBO?

No side effects have been found with SBO therapy, which appears to be remarkably safe. Therefore, I can recommend it for the following persons:

Anyone who has gastrointestinal symptoms such as gas, diarrhea, constipation, and heartburn.

One young male with Crohn's Disease tried many treatments for this disease but grew steadily worse until he weighed only 104 pounds. He started SBO and began to improve after one month. His weight steadily increased as his diarrhea waned and in one year he was back to 180 pounds.

A trial in celiac disease (non tropical sprue) and cystic fibrosis might be beneficial, as SBO appears to have strong capability to correct gastrointestinal symptoms. Both these conditions are associated with impaired absorption of nutrients from food.

Consider using in any disease of unknown cause for a trial period of two months. This group of diseases would include: amyotrophic lateral sclerosis, Creutzfeldt-Jacob disease (possible slow virus caused), sarcoidosis, ankylosing spondylitis and many others.

Consider using in any disease for which there is no known effective treatment. There would only be the expense of a two-month course of therapy.

Consider using in infectious diseases of viral, bacterial, fungal or parasitic origin.

Individual Immune Enhancement

Any individual who wants to improve his immune status and thus hopefully ward off bacterial and viral infections should consider taking SBO. Follow the dosage suggestions on the bottle.

SBO can be obtained from *Natural Health Team* 800-416-2806.

Bromelain

Bromelain is an enzyme made from pineapple that has anti-inflammatory actions. This will be discussed in more detail in Chapter 19.

A patient with ulcerative colitis read in *Dr. Whitaker's Health and Healing* that bromelain was an effective agent to stop inflammation. Ulcerative colitis is a serious inflammatory illness that causes thickening of the whole colon in severe cases and may eventuate into cancer after years of illness.

She was scheduled to have a colectomy, as this is effective in saving a patient's life but decided to try three 200 mg tablets of bromelain three times daily. Her condition steadily improved and the surgery was cancelled. Since this helped her, it could help others with this disease.

Cystic Fibrosis

Dr. Joel Wallach, in his book, *Let's Play Doctor*

(Double Happiness Company, Bonita, CA, 1996) reports he discovered that cystic fibrosis is a deficiency disease caused by selenium deficiency in the diet of the mother. Dr. Wallach states that cystic fibrosis can be prevented by supplying the mother with selenium *during* the pregnancy. He relates that cystic fibrosis can in some cases, be successfully treated by giving selenium to a child born with cystic fibrosis.

Ulcerative Colitis And Crohn's Disease

Ulcerative colitis is a serious colon disease that causes diarrhea, bloody stools, weight loss and may eventually lead to colon cancer in about 10% of cases. At times, an urgent removal of the whole colon is necessary to save a patient's life with this disorder.

Crohn's Disease is another serious diarrhea illness with recurring obstructions of the small bowel or colon that often require surgery. This condition may reappear after surgery and there may be associated fistulas to the rectal area, eye inflammation, specific skin rashes and arthritis in persons with this disease. Both of these disorders are reported to respond to Cetyl Myristolate (CM). Since therapy for both these diseases is often difficult, having a new approach could be very beneficial.

See Chapter 6 on Rheumatoid Arthritis for information about CM which is available from health food stores and our *Natural Health Team*.

Hemorrhoids

Hemorrhoids are simply varicose veins in the rectal area. During our lifetime approximately 50% of people will experience a problem with hemorrhoids. It is not unusual to have a clot form in one of these veins secondary to stagnant blood flow out of the vein.

These clots are frequently very painful at the site of the clot and surgeons are often needed to incise the painful swelling and remove the clot.

Hemorrhoids can also cause discomfort and itching. They may also bleed whenever the overlying distended vein ruptures. At times the hemorrhoid will protrude out through the anal opening. When they can no longer be easily replaced, surgery may be needed as may be the situation when bleeding is extensive.

For symptomatic hemorrhoids, white volcanic ash has been found to be an effective therapy. This clay contains no mercury, lead, preservatives, coloring, chemicals or sand. Dr. Victor Marcial-Vega relates that volcanic ash was successful in eliminating symptoms in 98 out of 100 consecutive cases. The two cases where improvement was not evident were both found to have cancer in the rectal area, which caused the hemorrhoids to appear.

A tube containing the volcanic ash is injected into the rectum initially and then repeated in one week.

This product is available from Health Horizons at 305- 442 1233 or 1800 771 0255. It is also available from our *Natural Health Team* 800-416-2806.

Dry Mouth

Saliva is an important protection for the mouth. The fluid washes away bacteria and when saliva is absent it is common to have rampant cavity formation. Many modern medicines cause *decreased* saliva production.

In a medical study at the Institute of Dentistry in Finland, researchers found out that 4% trimethylglycine (Betaine) added to toothpaste resolved the problem of dry mouth. This therapy can be obtained in health food stores. Avoid buying Betaine HCL as this is acidic and could cause burning in the mouth.

Be A Life Saver

I would encourage you to learn how to do the *Heimlich Maneuver*. Many people, particularly the elderly, are vulnerable to getting a piece of meat or food stuck in their throat. In this situation, the vocal cords will not work, so this person cannot speak and is obviously choking.

By placing your fist in the upper abdomen and then forcibly moving the fist toward the spine, great pressure is exerted on the esophagus and the bolus of food will usually pop out. If the first trial fails, use a little more force on the second. A 7-year-old child recently saved the life of a schoolmate because she knew how to do this.

Chapter 18

Anxiety, Depression And Behavioral Disturbances

Ten per cent of persons visiting physicians in the USA suffer from depression. This is a common problem. In Europe, St. John's Wort (SJW) is a widely used treatment for depression. *Up to 50% of persons diagnosed with depression in Germany are treated initially with SJW.* Long-term usage may cause sun sensitivity in fair skinned individuals *but there are no serious side effects.* A study of St. John's Wort showed that SJW *had fewer side effects than a placebo.*

SJW is believed to act by *prolonging* the effect of the mood enhancing brain chemical serotonin. There may also be prolongation of the action of dopamine and norepinephrine.

Drug interactions with cyclosporin, indivir, digoxin. theophylline and amitriptyline have been reported, so persons on those drugs should avoid St. John's Wort.

The SSRI antidepressants (Zoloft, Paxil, Prozac), the tricyclic antidepressants (Elavil, Tofranil) and monoamine oxidase inhibitors (Nardil, Parnate) all have some serious side effects. If you are taking any of the above, SJW should be used only after talking with your physician.

Having fewer side effects than a placebo and the absence of serious side effects after many years of use by millions of people means that SJW is a remarkably safe treatment.

The dose recommended is 300 mg twice daily of standardized herb containing .3% hypericin. St. John's Wort is widely available in health food stores and can be obtained from *Natural Health Team* 800-416-2806.

A second natural agent for treating depression is the herbal extract 5-hydroxytyptophan which is the direct precursor of serotonin. The dose is 100 mg three times daily.

SAME (s-adenyl-methionine) is another *natural* antidepressant. SAME is found in every cell in the body. This substance is a *natural* metabolite produced from the essential amino acid methionine and adenosine triphosphate (ATP). SAME is a precursor for glutathione, Coenzyme A, and taurine. This also boosts levels of serotonin and balances the levels of other neurotransmitters that are important in regulating mood.

This is the safest and most effective anti- depressant in the world. (SAME s-adenosylmethionine page 224 *Disease Prevention and Treatment, Expanded Third Edition)* published by The Life Extension Foundation, Hollywood, Florida.

Doses range from 400 to 1600 mg daily, but as little as 35mg daily has been used with favorable results. Obtain from health food stores.

Inositol

This substance is a B vitamin found in lecithin, brewer's yeast, liver, wheat germ, and whole grains. The body creates inisotol from glucose so it is always available.

Alzheimer's Disease

Recent research has suggested some new uses for inositol. It may improve language and orientation in Alzheimer's Disease patients given 6000 mg. daily.

Obsessive Compulsive Disorder

Patients taking 18 grams of inositol daily for 6 weeks exhibited significant improvement in symptoms of Obsessive Compulsive Disorder (Amer. Journal of Psychiatry vol. 153, page 1219-1221, 1996.)

Panic Disorder

Decrease in frequency and severity of panic attacks was observed after 4 weeks in individuals taking 12 grams of inositol daily (Amer. Journal of Psychiatry, vol. 152, page 1084-1086, 1995.)

Depression

Twelve persons with depression exhibited improvement in the Hamilton Depression Rating Scale after one month of 12 grams of inositol daily.

Inisotol is present in brain tissue in large amounts and functions in nerve communications. This functions as a backup system for regulating serotonin levels in the brain.

This may help persons who have failed to benefit from selective serotonin reuptake inhibitors (SSRI) and may also prove of value to those who have had side effects from SSRI therapy. Powdered packets of 4 grams and effervescent delivery systems are also available. Inositol is safe and readily available in health food stores and from *Natural Health Team* 800-416-2806.

Anxiety

Kava

Many individuals are in great stress in our modern society. Conventional psychoactive drugs have the problems of addiction and side effects.

Kava is a herbal preparation from the South Pacific that produces relaxation with no loss of mental acuity, thus making it an ideal supplement for today's frenetic lifestyle. This is a safe substance, reportedly free of side effects, and not addictive.

There is an actual enhancement of perception, awareness, and clarity of thought. This appears to have similar tranquilizing to benzodiazepines (Valium) without sedation. Beneficial effects can be seen in a week. The standard dose is 135 to 250 mg of 30% kavalactones three times daily for anxiety and two doses at bedtime as a sleep aid if needed.

Kava is available from BioBalance International, 888-246-4416.

New Therapy For Schizophrenia

Dr. Victor Marcial-Vega in his studies of NDF discovered that individuals with schizophrenia who took NDF often regained normal mental faculties after several months of NDF therapy. This suggests that NDF was removing some toxic agent from their bodies. When they experienced the return to normal mental function, they were able to discontinue NDF without relapse into a schizophenic condition.

We recommend that all schizophrenic persons consider a 6 month to 12 month trial of NDF. This therapy is far safer than the conventional phenothiazine drugs often used in the therapy of schizophrenia. The phenothiazine drugs can cause tardive dyskinessia which is a frequently permanent involuntary movement disorder, jaundice, bone marrow injury, low blood pressure and rarely an emergency loss of temperature control (neuroleptic malignant syndrome).

NDF can be obtained from Health Horizons 305-442 1233 or 800 771-0255 or from our *Natural Health Team* 800-416-2806.

Chapter 19

Acute And Chronic Musculoskeletal Pain Therapeutic Electro Membrane (TEM)

Millions of people seek relief from pain every day. *Acute* pain is defined as pain which results from an injury or trauma. This generally disappears. *Chronic* pain is a daily pain that lasts more than 6 months and often does not have a clearly defined (or treated) cause.

Some fundamental research by Dr. Robert Becker revealed that the pain response is *electrical,* not biochemical. This finding has been widely accepted and has led to the development of the TENS unit. (*Transcutaneous Electrical Nerve Stimulation*)

Electricity is now being widely used, for example, to stimulate healing of bone fracture in non-union areas of the bone. Electrical stimulation of muscle has also led to growth of muscle tissue in persons whose birth injury to the spinal cord had resulted in no muscle growth in the legs. Repair of the spinal injury was followed by inability to walk, due to failure of normal muscle development. After electrical muscle stimulation, these patients have regained almost full use of their limbs. The Canadian physicians are " tricking" these non- existent muscles into growing *by electrically causing muscle contractions, similar to those of strenuous exercise.* That, of course, builds those muscles.

Dr.Becker's research revealed that very low levels of current, in the range of 1 microampere, was adequate to achieve pain relief and stimulate healing. The amperage of the widely used TENS units is much higher, in the milli- ampere region. Dr. Becker believes that these *high* doses of current have 3 undesirable features.

1. The high current heats the tissues, which causes cell damage.

2. If metal electrodes are used, the positive electrode will give off ions of the metal used (stainless steel). These ions are quite toxic to the cells. These positive charged ions will be electrically repelled by the positive field of the electrode and will be driven some distance into the body.

3. With any level of high voltage, the water within the tissues is subjected to electrolysis, which breaks up the water molecule into gases like hydrogen, which is toxic to cells. High levels of voltage can kill all cells at the site.

Dr. Becker has found that much of the healing seen at the site of TENS application was actually the body's recovery from the injury of excessive electrical current. His experiments have consistently shown that *only very low* electrical currents are needed for healing.

The new units use below 500 milli-amperes, usually between 40 to 250, instead of TENS which uses from 1000 to 5000. Weak stimuli increase physiologic activity, whereas very strong stimuli inhibit or abolish activity (ARNDT-SCHULZ LAW).

Dr. N. Cheng found that weak currents increased ATP (an indicator of cellular energy levels) by up to 50%, but there was *no* increase when high currents were used. Furthermore, amino acid transport went up by 30 to 40% with low currents and was inhibited with high currents. *Clearly, lower current is better.*

A new product TEM (Therapeutic Electrical Membrane) has a low cost, is convenient, uses no electrodes, is safe and is as simple to use as applying a bandage.

Dr. Caoming of the Beijing Institute of Technology used a composition material capable of holding an electrical charge (electret). This was patented in 1986 and is widely used throughout the Orient .

The amperage used ranges from 5 to 10 microamperes. Injured tissue has an excess of positive ions and the TEM is negatively charged. An electrical circuit begins as soon as the patch is applied. The patch cannot be felt, as it is *below the sensibility level of sensory nerves.* These charges continue to flow until the membrane is completely discharged at 48 hours. If the pain relief and swelling are incompletely resolved at 48 hours, apply another patch.

Conditions that can be helped include chronic pain, contusions, sprains, strains, neck pain, finger arthritis, frozen shoulder, tennis elbow, backache, knee injuries, bursitis, knotted muscles, fractures, phlebitis, herpes zoster, mastitis, swelling and inflammation. *Favorable results are seen in approximately 90% of acute problems and 85% of chronic problems.*

The patches can be cut with plastic scissors to fit small injuries. Keep the patches dry (cover with a protective plastic membrane or remove before showering). These have a shelf life of 5 years. The patches are available in packets of 5, 10, and 20 patches.

We feel that keeping a five or ten patch packet should be ideal for a family to keep available for unexpected accidents and injuries.

Obtain from Professional Products Co., 120 S. 16th Ave. Brighton, CO or from our *Natural Health Team* 800-416-2806.

Chapter 20

Asthma, Hay Fever, Chronic Sinusitis, Recurring Ear Infections In Infants And Emphysema

Dr. Lon Jones of Hale Center, Texas became very concerned about his small granddaughter's recurring ear infections. Dr. Jones knew that research in Finland (a very advanced medical country) had shown that a sugar (xylitol) chewing gum had reduced ear infections by 40% in children when it was given 8 times daily to prevent caries. Dr. Jones reasoned that if xylitol gum could cut ear infections by 40%, good things might happen if a solution of xylitol was inhaled into the upper nasal passages.

Xylitol has the interesting property that it causes bacteria on the surface of a membrane to become dislodged so they can be washed away.

To his great surprise and pleasure, he discovered that not only did infantile ear infections cease *but chronic sinus infections; allergic rhinitis, bronchitis and asthma were eliminated.*

It is important that the atomizer is used correctly. A child should be on its back when the solution is placed in each nostril. Adults should stare at their feet. Then inject one spray toward the back of your head and one spray toward the top of your head on each side. Do this three or four times daily until symptoms start to subside.

People with severe cases of asthma should use the spray every one to two hours for two or three days, when the dose frequency can be cut back to two or three times daily.

The favorable response of infantile ear infections, bronchitis, asthma, hay fever, and chronic sinus infections to such a simple measure as washing bacteria out of the upper nasal passages *suggests that colonization of bacteria in the upper nasal airways may be playing an important role in causing these conditions.* This washing away of bacteria has no metabolic effect on bacteria and *resistant bacteria are not created.*

I would like to tell you my personal experience with Xlear. For eight or nine years I have been bothered by right frontal headaches three or four days weekly on awakening. There had been morning postnasal drainage and morning cough daily. Two or three times yearly I would develop profuse post nasal drainage that rapidly became yellow. At the same time I would develop severe coughing with sputum, wheezing, and fever. Often antibiotics had to be taken before recovery would begin.

After four days on Xlear, the morning headaches disappeared along with the postnasal drainage and coughing. Xlear appears to have stopped my chronic sinusitis and recurring bronchitis. I continue to use it daily.

This product can be obtained from XLEAR 877- 332 1001 and from *Natural Health Team* 800-416-2806.

Bromelain

Another product to consider for asthma is bromelain which has anti-inflammatory activity. There is an inflammatory component to the asthmatic attack. Use of bromelain during an acute attack, 600 mg three time's daily could be effective in some persons. It can be taken in a small maintenance dosage of 200 mg two or three times daily to help prevent further attacks. As with most natural health solutions, it will do no harm.

Bromelain can be obtained from health food stores and from *Natural Health Team* 800-416-2806.

Emphysema

Cetyl myristolate (CM) has been used in emphysema and related lung disorders with great improvement. The scar tissue remains, but the volume of inspired air may increase by up to 35%. Progression of the emphysema stops. *These are dramatic results.*

Smokers who quit cigarettes may see a 10% to 15% improvement in breathing. *Emphysema is widely believed to be a progressive disease, so any therapy that stops progression is extremely valuable.*

Cetyl Myristolate is available from Brower Enterprises 800 373 6067 and from *Natural Health Team* 800-416-2806.

Sarcoidosis

Sarcoidosis is a disease of unknown cause that is more common in Afro-Americans than Caucasians. The disease causes nodules and scarring in the involved organs. The disease is often discovered by a routine chest x-ray in an adult with no symptoms. The lung is the most common organ involved in the disease, but the eyes, skin, bones and joints may be involved.

Lung symptoms may include cough, shortness of breath and wheezing. When the lung symptoms are advanced or the disease involves critical structures (eyes, nervous system) cortisone therapy is usually effective. Often it is impossible to discontinue cortisone which may need to be maintained in low dosage.

Because of the clear benefits of cetyl myristolate in stopping the progression of emphysema and other inflammatory diseases, we think that one month of CM in two capsules, three times daily, could be helpful. This should prove safer than long-term steroid therapy if it succeeds.

Chapter 21

Urinary Tract Infections And Kidney Stones

Mannitol For Recurring Urinary Tract Infections

Resuming the theme of bacteria being washed away from surfaces, we can proceed to mannitol. This is another natural sugar that is able to dislodge bacteria from the bladder and lead to cessation of urinary infections for many individuals.

Mannitol is readily absorbed after ingestion, but most is not metabolized, so it has *no effect* on blood sugar levels. Research studies have shown that mannitol is 10 times more active against e.coli (the agent causing 80% of urinary infections) than the fructose in cranberry juice.

Recurring urinary infections are common in patients with impaired emptying of the bladder from prostate enlargement, some sexually active women and many individuals with blocked drainage of the urinary tract. Antibiotic drugs have not proven to be an ideal solution for urinary tract infections for the following reasons:

- Using an antibiotic may create bacterial organisms that no longer respond to the usual antibiotics (bacterial resistance). This is particularly dangerous if there is impaired drainage of the urinary tract. What may occur then is that an infection with e. coli, which is usually not very destructive to the kidney, may become converted to an infection with pseudomonas, proteus, or another very pathogenic bacteria, which is capable of destroying a kidney in a year and very hard to eradicate with conventional antibiotics.

- If there is obstruction of the urinary tract, it is nearly impossible to sterilize the urine. What happens then is that the antibiotic used simply kills all the urinary bacteria that are sensitive to it, leaving a predominance of the organisms that were not killed by it. These are invariably more dangerous to the kidneys and much harder to impossible to eradicate. For this reason physicians may wish to hold off on antibiotics until the obstruction can be simultaneously corrected by surgery.

- I was always pleased to find e.coli in the urine in elderly men and women, as they were less likely to destroy kidney tissue. If there was no fever or kidney pain it appeared sensible to leave the patient untreated, particularly if it was impossible to correct an obstruction.

- The availability of this *natural* technique to manage urinary tract infections could turn out to be very opportune.

- *The urine bacteria are simply flushed out in the urine along with the mannitol.* Mannitol is absorbed in the upper gastrointestinal tract and thus does not disturb the intestinal flora. There are no side effects.

Since this technique does not cause a metabolic effect on the urinary bacteria, hopefully no resistance to antibiotics will develop. The usual dose is 1/2 teaspoon of mannitol every three hours for 24 to 48 hours, when improvement is expected and the dosage can be reduced to four times daily. For infections related to sexual intercourse, taking 1/2 teaspoon one hour before and 1/2 teaspoon after sexual relations is effective.

Severe kidney infections (pyelonephritis) take two to three days to clear and may need a daily maintenance of 1/2 teaspoon daily. In severe kidney infections the mannitol should be taken every two hours for the first two days. The d-mannitol has a sweet taste and can be mixed with juice, milk, or water. *D-mannitol is effective for 80% of urine infections.*

Mannitol can be purchased from Bio-Tech Pharmacal at 800-345 1199 or our *Natural Health Team* 800-416-2806.

Kidney Stones

Kidney stones are common and often are associated with severe pain.

A natural product called chancra piedra (CP) has been useful in helping patients expel kidney stones. It is a very effective antispasmodic, which relaxes the smooth muscle in the ureter, which connects the kidney to the bladder. This relaxation permits the stone to pass down the ureter and out of the bladder, unless it is quite large.

Larger stones can often be broken or extracted by a urologist. For stones that a urologist is unable to remove, lithotripter therapy can smash the stone into powder or small particles that are easily passed. The lithotripter is an ingenious German development that uses shock waves of high frequency sound to safely smash the stones.

Dr. Wolfram Wieman of Nuremburg, Germany reviewed 100 cases of kidney stones treated with chancra piedra *and found 94% of those with smaller to normal size stones were able to pass the stone.*

Any person who has a stone has a good possibility of having another. Chancra piedra has been found to be effective in preventing the accumulation of calcium oxalate crystals, which represent the start of a new stone. There appears to be a component in the CP that prevents stones from forming. The dose is 30 drops, one or two times a day. CP prevents new stones, *even in the presence of high levels of calcium oxalate in the urine.*

CP can be purchased from Raintree Nutrition, 800-780 5902. It is also available from our *Natural Health Team* 800-416-2806.

Chapter 22

Inflammatory Illnesses

Conditions characterized by marked swelling and inflammation are experienced by almost everyone in life. This includes insect, scorpion, bee, wasp and snakebites. Poisonous snakebites may have such massive swelling that there can be grave danger of amputation because of impaired circulation from the pressure of the massive swelling on arteries.

Also to be considered are fractured bones, which if large like the hip, may have an enormous amount of swelling. Dental conditions at times may have considerable swelling. Severe sunburn frequently has marked swelling.

The final category is ulcerative colitis in which the inflammatory reaction may extend through the whole width of the colon. The use of 900 mg of bromelain three times daily saved a patient with severe ulcerative colitis from total colectomy surgery. (See Chapter 17 Gastrointestinal Diseases)

The treatment, which might be beneficial in these conditions, is bromelain. Bromelain is an enzyme extracted from pineapple, which has powerful anti-inflammatory activity in high dosage. Bromelain is often given to arthritic patients to help curtail the inflammatory reaction. Bromelain also prevents clumping of platelets, which may help ward off blood clots.

In patients who have trouble digesting their food, bromelain when taken with meals, helps break up proteins, fats, and carbohydrates *and thus may improve digestion.*

This is not expensive and it could be a good therapy to keep around the house in your medicine cabinet, as one cannot plan falls, sprains, bites and accidents.

My personal experience converted me into a strong believer. Recently I declined a root canal and had the removal of a molar, which took one and one half hours. The dentist was obviously fatigued and he admitted to me that it was one of the most difficult extractions he had ever experienced. On arrival at home, the anesthesia was still present. I started 600 mg of bromelain three times daily and *did not have either pain or swelling of the face, which greatly surprised the dentist.* The anti swelling properties of this natural product seem to be substantial for a myriad of problems, which cause swelling and inflammation.

See Chapter 20 for more information about the use of bromelain in asthma.

Bromelain is available from health food stores and from *Natural Health Team.* 800-416-2806.

Chapter 23

Arteriosclerosis And Varicose Veins

When I attended medical school we were taught that when your arteries were narrowed and blocking off your life was over and that you would soon die. Today, of course, this is no longer believed.

Dr. Blankenhorn at the University of Southern California Medical School did some extremely important studies about 15 years ago. He performed arteriograms on the main artery to the leg (Femoral Artery) in patients with narrowed arteries. These patients were then placed on an intensive program to help their arteries (quit cigarettes, eat a low fat diet, lower cholesterol with medicine, and bring the blood pressure under control with medicine).

One year later, the arteriograms of the Femoral Artery were repeated. Some patients got worse, some stayed the same *but a surprising number showed improvement.*

This same type study in the coronary artery system has confirmed that bad coronary arteries to the heart can get better. This tells us that *the circulatory system is dynamic and a changed lifestyle can be very beneficial.*

Aromatherapy For Leg Ulcers, Non -Healing Wounds And Incisions

Impaired circulation of blood often leads to non-healing leg ulcers. There are two general forms of leg ulcers (arteriosclerotic and varicose). The arteriosclerotic ulcers are caused by poor circulation secondary to narrowed arteries in the aorta or leg.

The tissue level of oxygen is so low that any minor trauma to the leg will produce an expanding non-healing ulceration. These are often painful.

At times it is possible to improve the circulation by coring out the tissue obstructing the arterial channel or by bypassing the obstructed area with a graft.

Frequently diabetes plays an important role in these ulcers. Diabetics have frequent problems with accelerated narrowing of both large and small arteries as well as great difficulty fighting off bacterial infections. These ulcerations often heal very slowly if they can be healed at all. They become a source of great disability with long stays in hospitals and nursing homes as well as surgeries to clear the ulcer from infection and try to restore better blood flow.

Venous (varicose) ulcers are caused by long standing swelling of the legs secondary to loss of valves in the veins and obstruction to the flow of blood out of leg veins secondary to clots (thrombi) in the veins. Following a clot in a major leg vein it is not unusual to have permanent swelling of the leg. When this progresses ulceration may appear above the ankle on the inner side of the leg.

About 20% of people have problems with varicose veins. They are five times more common in women than men and often begin during pregnancy, Approximately 15% of individuals with problem varicose veins have a family history of varicose veins.

When the blood stagnates in the legs due to faulty valves and the dependent status of the legs there is failure to return fluid to the circulation and very impaired oxygenation of the leg tissue. When an ulcer begins it is frequently difficult to heal and successful healing often is followed by reappearance of the ulcer at a later date.

For these problems in healing we suggest a trial of aromatherapy with the essential oil lavender. *Aromatic plant oils are some of the most powerful antioxidants known.*

They also eradicate virus, fungi, bacteria and parasites. For this reason, essential oils remain fresh and sterile in a bottle for more than 30 years.

They assist in detoxification by breaking down hydrocarbons, such as petrochemicals and chemical pesticides, into carbon dioxide and water through the promotion of ozone formation in the environment that they are infused into.

Lavender oil appears to accomplish healing by building up the nutritional state of the cells in the base of the ulcer and by killing all fungi, parasites and bacteria encountered in the ulcer (oxygen from ozone kills these organisms).

The lavender oil is supplied sterile in 1/8-ounce bottles. The aroma oil is applied by tapping the overturned bottle so that drops will come out on the ulcer one at a time. Removed of dead tissue on the surface of the ulcer is not necessary. Do not cover the ulcer with a dressing.

Dr. Vega relates that this is always curative without scar formation. Lavendar Essential Oil can be obtained from Health Horizons 900 981 7157 or from our *Natural Health Team* 800-416-2806.

Strokes

Strokes are a common cause of death. There are 3 major categories of strokes.

Cerebral Hemorrage

This is often a catastrophic event in which rupture of an artery within the brain tissue causes sudden grave symptoms. The patient may develop paralysis, collapse and coma. Hypertension may be the major reason for the ruptured blood vessel and this can be made less likely to occur by good control of blood pressure in hypertensive patients.

Ruptured Berry Aneurysm

A different form of hemorrhage is the rupture of an abnormal artery, which was weak from birth. This condition may be associated with other diseases and, at times, arteriograms in patients' relatives will uncover a weak artery (aneurysm) which can be repaired surgically. The rupture of this type aneurysm causes a severe headache.

Cerebral Thrombosis

Thrombosis of a cerebral artery or embolism of a cerebral artery. A thrombosis affects an artery which has been partially occluded by arteriosclerosis. An embolism is a blood clot carried by the blood stream from either the neck arteries or the heart to the brain. These pieces of cholesterol and clotted blood land in cerebral arteries, causing death of adjacent brain tissue. This is identical to the injury produced by a clot in a cerebral artery.

At times, badly narrowed arteries produce symptoms of insufficient blood supply and the patient can be started on medicine to prevent blood clotting, or the narrowed artery can have the cholesterol plaques reamed out.

However, this type surgery has recently been shown to have an 11% incidence of either death or a new stroke in the 30 day period following surgery, so caution might be wise before proceeding with this type operation.

Hyperbaric Oxygen

When a stroke occurs, Dr. Julian Whitaker has seen remarkable improvement in patients' symptoms by going to a hyperbaric oxygen chamber where oxygen is administered under pressure. This system of administering oxygen appears to allow healing of areas of brain tissue that are suffering from a lack of oxygen.

One patient was carried into Dr. Whitaker's office two weeks after a stroke. Following two weeks of hyperbaric oxygen treatment *she walked out of the hospital.*

A second patient suffered severe speech, vision and hearing deficits after a stroke and was confined to a wheel chair. Six months later he went to a hyperbaric center for therapy. Three weeks later he could walk with only slight residual balance problems. This is a form of treatment that has no danger and if you have a favorable response, it is well worth the effort to locate a hyperbaric chamber.

DMSO is a potent solvent often used to facilitate the movement of topical therapies through the skin. The actions of DMSO that make it valuable in a stroke are:

- Anti- inflammatory activity

- Anti swelling

- Prevents clotting of blood

- Diuretic effect to remove fluid collecting at the site of the stroke.

- Hypothermic action

- Vasodilatation increases blood flow

- Stimulates respiration

- Crosses the blood brain barrier, which blocks many agents from being effective in a stroke setting.

- Corrects membrane instability

In a study at the Mayo Clinic, 26 monkeys were split into two groups.

One of the main arteries to the brain was clamped for 17 hours.

Half the monkeys received DMSO and the other half got no treatment. When the brain was studied 7 days later, there was significant protection from severe damage seen in the monkeys that did get DMSO.

Unfortunately these important results have not been followed up by use of DSMO in strokes. An individual suffering from small strokes might end up with much less permanent brain damage by application of 70% DSMO with 30% distilled water to the skin once or twice daily.

DMSO is available from Omaha Vaccine. However, be aware that studies are still underway to determine if it will ever be approved for human use.

Intermittent Claudication

Arteriosclerosis is generally a process that involves arteries in all parts of the body. When the arteries in the distal aorta and legs are seriously blocked, the condition is called intermittent claudication. This problem is associated with pain in leg muscles after exertion, and impotence. If the exertion is continued, the pain gets progressively worse until walking is impossible.

With rest, an adequate amount of blood is again delivered to the leg muscles so that walking can be resumed. Surgical repair of the narrowed aorta or leg arteries may lead to better leg circulation and subsidence of the exertional pain. There has never been a good medicine for intermittent claudication until recently.

A natural substance from Tibet named Padma Basic contains 20 herbs. In 1985 researchers studied Padma Basic and found that *persons on this treatment were able to have a 100% increase in the distance they could walk before pain appeared, after 16 weeks of therapy..* (Schweiz Med Wochenschr 115(22): 752-756, 1985). Padma Basic was well tolerated.

Three further studies have confirmed these findings.

Padma does not work by vasodilation. The compound is a powerful anti-oxidant and benefits blood lipids with falls in both cholesterol and triglyceride values. Platelet clumping is also decreased, making the blood less likely to clot.

Anyone with intermittent claudication should be encouraged to walk long distances daily, as the persistent need for more blood flow to meet the muscles' exertional needs over a period of time leads to the development of new small vessels in the muscles, which can decrease claudication. Walk until pain appears and then rest until it stops, before you resume walking.

A common problem called "restless legs" is also benefited by Padma. Persons with this condition have constant leg movement at night. Some cases relate to metabolic abnormality in calcium or acid base balance, but most are felt to be caused by poor leg circulation. Two to four weeks of Padma will often resolve this problem.

Because improvement in walking with Padma Basic often takes 4 weeks to be noticeable, my suggestion would be that you take Padma Basic for two months and then observe the effect before taking more. It is not harmful.

The dosage for adults is two tablets three times daily before meals. Children over three years take 1 tablet three times daily. Below three years, the dose is ½ tablet three times daily. Padma is painstakingly manufactured to be free of pesticides and contaminants. The shelf life is 5 years.

Padma Basic is obtainable from Nutri Center USA 800-701 8648 and from our *Natural Health Team* 800-416-2806.

Profibe

Dr. James Cerda of the University of Florida Medical School tested a compound of natural citrus pectin in experimental pigs, which had very elevated cholesterol levels. Giving these animals citrus pectin was associated with striking decreases in the degree of arteriosclerosis found.

In humans treated with citrus pectin, there was an average cholesterol fall of 21mg. and a 21% fall in LDL as well. HDL and triglycerides were not altered. Possibly quercetin from the flavinoids in grapefruit is causing less oxidation of LDL cholesterol. This compound appears to be a safe way to help the arteries for those persons with arteriosclerosis. Again, it is a natural product with no known harmful effects to the body.

The citrus pectin product is called ProFibe and can be obtained from CerBurg Products Ltd. 800-756 3999

Varicose Veins

Enlarged veins (varicose veins) that may become painful and the source for blood clots are common in women after multiple pregnancies, obese patients and in some families. Damaged valves in the veins cause increased pressure in the veins and impaired return of blood from the veins to the heart.

This stagnant blood in these veins is more likely to clot (phlebitis). Additionally, there is impaired return of blood from the extremities and chronic swelling of the legs (edema) often appears. At times, the circulation is so impaired that nutrition of the skin is inadequate and ulcers may appear (varicose ulcers).

A *natural* therapy that improves the tone in the veins has been used for years. This is derived from the seeds of the horse chestnut. The resulting improved tone leads to a *decrease* in the edema fluid and lessened discomfort from the enlarged veins.

Another measure that helps is the wearing of tight elastic stockings. If clotting occurs, anticoagulant therapy may be needed.

Horse chestnut is available in health food stores. This therapy has been widely used in Germany for many years.

Chapter 24

High Cholesterol (Hypercholesterolemia)

What About Cholesterol?

Cholesterol is needed in every cell of the body as it is the chemical precursor from which the body produces bile acids, provitamin D3 and many vital hormones. The body can make cholesterol whether there is any cholesterol in the diet or not. By removing all cholesterol from the diet, the blood cholesterol will only fall by about 20% to 25%. Cholesterol is dissolved and kept in solution as a flowing liquid when there are adequate amounts of essential fatty acids. The melting point of cholesterol, where it would deposit on artery walls, is 300 degrees F. When lecithin is present, the melting point of cholesterol falls to 180 degrees where it is still insoluble.

However, when the essential fatty acids linoleic and linolenic are present in sufficient quantity, the melting point of cholesterol falls to 32 degrees below normal body temperature. Even in the presence of an arterial injury, cholesterol will have a more difficult time depositing with platelets on the injured artery wall because the essential fatty acids have made the blood more fluid.

Many factors are involved in the creation of the arteriosclerotic plaque, which precedes a heart attack or stroke problem. Among these are:

- Hypercholesterolemia The best proof of the cholesterol level being a risk factor for arterial damage is the genetic disorder of Familial Hypercholesterolemia. This occurs in about one out of every 500 persons. These persons have severe artery disease at a young age, which is greatly worsened by smoking.

- Homocysteinemia Persons with elevated levels of homocysteine are at risk for arteriosclerosis. This can and should be corrected with adequate amounts of folic acid, B 12, pyridoxine, and trimethylglycine. The only way you can be sure you are getting adequate amount of therapy is to regularly monitor blood levels of homocysteine. Current estimates are that 30 to 40% of arterial disease is related to high levels of homocysteine.

The statin groups of cholesterol-lowering drugs have been effective, but with the predominant side effects being abnormal liver function tests in a few patients and rare cases of skeletal muscle necrosis (injury) and death. Baycol, a major cholesterol-lowering drug was withdrawn in August 2001 due to the relative high incidence of death of users. Powerful chemical substances often help the specific problem they're created for, but can have long-term harmful effects, which may not become known for years. The frequency of recent drug recalls is proof of this.

The availability of *natural* substances like food (flax oil) to lower cholesterol suggests that these natural products might be able to safely replace the more expensive statin drugs.

In most cases natural solutions are harmless when taken properly. Not all natural products will do everything we expect for every person, since every person is unique. *The ones we have chosen will generally work in many cases and in most cases will do no harm.*

Where Do Fish Oils Fit In?

There is a well- documented inverse relationship between the amount of cold-water fish eaten and the occurrence of arteriosclerosis of the heart arteries (CAD).

Dr. Dyerberg of Denmark did a fascinating study of Greenland Eskimos, which showed that the high fat intake of whale, seal, and walrus meat was counteracted by a very high intake of cold- water fish.

One community of 2,000 persons, which were followed for 10 years, did not have a single death from a heart attack.

Cold-water fish contain large amounts of Omega 3 fatty acids in the form of eicosapentaenoic acid (EPA) and docosahexaenoic (DHA) acid.

These fish oils have a wonderful ability to keep arteries open. They also lower cholesterol, lower triglycerides, prevent clotting of blood, lower blood pressure, and improve arthritis.

Dr. Kromhaut of Holland studied dietary habits of 852 middle aged men. The men eating high amounts of fish had only 36% of the risk of dying from heart artery disease of those who ate no fish.

There are two problems that seem to hinder wider use of fish oil.

Can you be sure the fish were caught in the ocean, instead of grown on a fish farm where their food is grain not omega 3 marine precursors? Large, long- lived ocean fish, like tuna and swordfish, have mercury.

Smaller ocean fish such as salmon, anchovies, mackerel, halibut, whitefish, mahi mahi, haddock, cod and scrod are fine. Some lake trout and catfish have industrial pollutants (polychlorinated biphenyls).

When eating fish, cut out the dark fatty portions, as these are the sites where pollutants are stored.

Several natural treatments to correct high cholesterol (hypercholesterolemia) will be discussed in this chapter.

Inositol Hexaniacinate (IHN)

Conventional niacin lowers cholesterol levels and relieves symptoms of Raynaud's Syndrome. This vitamin has serious side effects (facial flushing and gastrointestinal distress), which are avoided in the inositol formulation.

Inositol hexaniacinate (INH) is a niacin precursor that lowers cholesterol and triglycerides and raises HDL. The cholesterol precursor VLDL is decreased by the liver in the presence of INH. This results in lower cholesterol. The cold hands seen in Raynaud's Syndrome are warmed and circulation in leg arteries may benefit from IHN. The dose should start at 500 mg to 1000 mg. daily and can be increased to 2500 mg daily if necessary. Physician monitoring for liver cell injury and for elevation of blood sugar is needed in diabetic patients who can get high sugar values on niacin treatment.

Inositol hexaniacinate can be obtained in many health food stores and from *Natural Health Team* 800-416-2806.

Turmeric Spice or Curcumin

(one of the components of curry that gives it a yellow color and a distinctive odor is called curcumin). Doses of 500 mg daily of turmeric were followed by a 11.6% fall in cholesterol and a rise in HDL of 29% within 7 days, when administered to persons with high cholesterol values.

Researchers in Taiwan confirmed these findings with 500 mg of curcumin daily and also noted a prevention of restenosis after balloon angioplasty using curcumin.

This can be found in the spice section of supermarkets and possibly health food stores.

Dimethylglycine (DMG)

(Chapter 2) has been used by several cardiologists with *unexpected* benefits. The dose of 125 mg daily dropped cholesterol and triglyceride levels, lowered blood pressure in hypertensive patients, reduced or stopped anginal pain and improved the patients physical and mental well being. This can be purchased from Wholesome Nutrition at Saratoga, CA. Phone 800-325 2664

Gugulipid (GLD)

This is a resin of the commiphora mukul tree of India. In one study of 125 patients, after 4 weeks of GLD there was an 11% decrease in cholesterol, a 16.8% drop in triglycerides, and a *60% increase in HDL.*

Raising the HDL by 1 mg. is believed to decrease the risk of heart attack by 2%. In another study from India, in 40 patients with hyperlipidmia after 12 weeks of Gugulipid there were 22% falls in cholesterol, 27% falls in triglycerides and a 36% rise in HDL.

These rises in HDL are extraordinary and, if valid, very important. I would suggest getting a full lipid panel (cholerestorol, HDL, LDL and tryglyceride) before and 6 weeks after treatment.

Gugulipid can be obtained from Nature's Distributors 800-6247114

Red Yeast

Red yeast is a spice used to prepare Peking Duck. Red yeast contains a family of compounds called statins. One of these statins is lovastatin (MEVACOR), a widely used drug to lower cholesterol. There are several other statins sold by pharmaceutical firms (Lipitor,Pravachol. Zocor, Baycol, Lescol). All these lower cholesterol.

Physicians experienced in natural medicine always prefer to use the whole plant rather than isolate one of it's parts as there is likely to be less side effects, making this safer for long term usage. With red yeast you are getting the whole compound, rather than a statin selected out of red yeast.

This means that you have a low blood level of many different statins instead of a very high blood level of one statin, as occurs in the pharmaceutical preparations.

Several studies have been performed on Monascus purpureus (Red Yeast Rice) showing effective cholesterol reduction. At Tufts University School of Medicine, 233 patients who took red yeast experienced an average 38-point drop in cholesterol over 8 weeks, with no side effects. In a study at UCLA, Dr. David Heber showed that red yeast led to a 17% reduction in cholesterol in 8 weeks, again with no side effects.

Natures Distributors (see gugulipid above) has a formulation of red yeast combined with gugulipid. This can also be obtained from *Natural Health Team*.

The suggested dose is three tablets daily with the evening meal. Persons taking Red Yeast or pharmaceutical statins should take 60 mg. of CoQ10 gel daily, as this substance becomes depleted on statin therapy.

Also monitoring of serial liver function results by a physician is necessary, as an occasional patient on statins or red yeast develops liver function abnormalities. The appearance of unexplained muscle tenderness (necrosis) may rarely occur with statins or red yeast therapy and calls for *immediate cessation of either treatment.*

Garlic

A liquid garlic extract from *Kyolic* caused a 12 to 31% fall in cholesterol in most subjects after 6 months. *Garlic also inhibits the oxidation of cholesterol, which is a key step in the creation of an arteriosclerotic plaque. The endothelial lining of blood vessels appears to be protected against oxidative damage.*

Garlic also inhibits platelet clumping and thus may aid in preventing blood clots. Garlic products are available in most health food stores.

Fish Oil

Hypertriglceridemia was reduced by 35% in persons taking fish oil (OMEGA 3 fatty acids).

Fiber

High intakes of fiber have shown slight lowering of cholesterol.

Green Tea

A study from Japan showed that intake of 9 cups of green tea in men was associated with lower cholesterol than in persons consuming only 2 cups daily.

Artichoke Leaf

An extract of artichoke leaves has also shown cholesterol and triglyceride lowering by about 12% . The dosage suggested is 300 mg, three times daily.

Flaxseed

Flaxseed contains large quantities of fiber. This fiber binds with bile acids in the intestine, which interferes with the re-absorption of cholesterol from the gut *causing considerable cholesterol to pass out with the stools.*

Use of ¼ cup (4 tablespoons) of ground flaxseed daily is enough. This can be placed in cereal, mixed with fruit in yogurt or cottage cheese or placed in salads. Substantial falls in cholesterol have been known to result.

This use of flaxseed is safe and accomplishes many other worthwhile health changes as well as its beneficial effect on cholesterol.

Flaxseed is available from many health food stores and *Natural Health Team* 800-416-2806.

There are 8 forms of Vitamin E. Four of these are tocopherols and four are tocotreinols. The tocopherols are powerful antioxidants but have no effect on cholesterol. The tocotrienols are up to 60 times more powerful as antioxidants and have the added benefit of lowering cholesterol as well as decreases the clotting of blood.

Vitamin E attaches to LDL cholesterol and prevents the oxidation of LDL cholesterol by free radicals. Only after LDL is oxidized is it able to injure the wall of the artery. Research at the UC Berkeley in 1991 disclosed that d-alpha tocotrienol had between 40 and 60 times higher antioxidant action than did conventional Vitamin E (tocopherol).

The tocotrienol form of Vitamin E has the same type of beneficial effect on blood clotting as that found in aspirin. The production of a powerful clotting substance (thromboxane A 2) is inhibited by up to 30% and platelet clumping is blocked by between 15 and 30%. No ulceration or gastrointestinal distress is found in tocotrienol therapy.

The effective statin cholesterol lowering drugs act by filling receptor sites that receive the cholesterol production stimulating enzyme HMG-CoA reductase. When this does not land on the receptor site the level of cholesterol in the blood falls. To overcome this blockage the body secretes great and greater quantities of HMG-CoA reductase, as much as 200 times the normal. Some authorities believe this excessive production of HMG-Co reductase may be the cause for liver injury that can occur with statin therapy. Tocotrienol E lowers the cholesterol nearly as well as the statins with no side effects. The action of Tocotrienol E causes destruction of HMG-CoA before it reaches the receptor sites.

Tocotrienol E is derived from rice bran oil. Decreases of cholesterol may range from 7% to 48% with average falls of 16%. The tocotrienol E is available as *Care Diem* from Aspen Nutritional Products 800 539 5195

Chapter 25

Longevity (A Tale Of 3 Healthy Older People)

Paul Bragg was the founder of the health food store industry in the United States. He was an expert in the field of good nutrition. *At age 95 he died when struck by a boat propeller while swimming in the ocean.*

I had the good fortune to meet his daughter Patricia about 15 years ago. She was the picture of radiant good health with light brown hair, a beautiful complexion, and a perfect figure. After some mental calculations it occurred to me she was almost certainly about 65. She looked 45.

The third person is Dr. Joanna Budwig mentioned in Chapter 14. *She is actively practicing medicine at age 95. These three persons illustrate the extreme importance of what we eat.*

The Braggs eat a proper amount of nutritious food. This is mixed with days of fasting. Dr. Budwig has eaten a flax based diet from childhood, which sounds close to vegetarian. Some authorities believe that flax is nature's most perfect food.

We have not been "programmed" to die at age 65 to 70. Premature deaths may be caused by what we do to our bodies. Dispensing with *artificial* foods (white flour, margarine, salad oils, shortenings, white rice, white sugar, carbonated beverages, frying) and curtailing excessive dietary protein, along with a marked increase in consumption of vegetables, fruit, fish, flax oil, and fiber could bring very beneficial changes in our health and add years to our lives.

This needs to be combined with drinking water that is not contaminated with fluoride, chlorine, heavy metals, pesticides, chemical wastes, petrochemicals, and infectious agents.

Taking proper vitamins, antioxidants, and minerals is also very rewarding.

Many individuals would like to live longer and remain healthy as they age, if this is possible. Glutathione (GTH) is an essential amino acid found in every cell in the body. Deficiency of this amino acid has long been known to be associated with the appearance of cataracts in the eye.

GTH is a very powerful antioxidant. Many human diseases are believed to be caused by cellular damage from *environmental* substances that affect everyone. These are:

AIR POLLUTION (cigarette smoke, smoke from the industrial burning of coal and oil and exhaust from vehicles).

POLLUTION OF DRINKING WATER with pesticides, chlorine, lead and heavy metals, petrochemical residue, fluoride, and infectious organisms.

FOOD POLLUTION Frying, grilling, and blackening food along with the widespread use of synthetic partially hydrogenated oils in salad dressings and margarine creates toxic free radicals that are difficult for the body to destroy. The long term exposure to free radicals is believed to cause the degenerative diseases that lead to death (malignancies, arteriosclerosis, arthritis and diabetes).

These three forms of pollution are constantly releasing free radicals that injure cells.

In a real sense, our immune systems are in a battle for our survival from the day we are born.

The antioxidants glutathione, Vitamin C, Vitamin E, Selenium and others are critical in preventing deterioration of our bodies. Some of these pollutants are unavoidable but others are self-induced, often by what we eat.

A research project in Spain discovered some important data. Frogs were given glutathione (GTH) along with substances believed to prolong the effect of GTH. These frogs were compared to frogs not getting GTH. At 14 months, 91% of the frogs getting GHT were alive compared to 46% of those not given GTH. When the GTH was stopped at 26 months, the survival rate of the remaining frogs plummeted.

Obviously, GTH is important in longevity. This experiment marked the first in which a *vertebrate animal's life was prolonged by taking antioxidants.*

Healthy individuals who have reached age 80 or more all have very high levels of glutathione in their blood. Persons with elevated levels of GTH in their blood stay healthy, while persons with hypertension, arthritis, heart disease, and diabetes all have low levels of GTH. (Dr. Calvin Lang and Dr. Mara Julius Journal Clinical Epidemiology 94: 47[9]: 1021-6)

How Can We Keep Our Glutathione Levels High?

Eat lots of cruciferous vegetables, which contain glutathione. This group includes Brussels sprouts, cauliflower, broccoli, cabbage, kale, bok choy, cress, mustard, horseradish, turnips, rutabagas, and kohlrabi. These same vegetables contain indole-3-carbinol that inactivates estrogen. *This may explain why persons eating these vegetables have a lower incidence of cancer of the breast, prostate, lungs, esophagus, bladder and especially the colon.*

Tests to measure GTH blood levels are very difficult to do because GTH is quickly oxidized when exposed to light, heat, and air.

There is controversy about how to raise GTH blood levels. In an experiment on seven normal persons taking 3000 mg. of GTH daily, there was no increase in blood levels after 7 days of therapy.

Supplements other than GTH may help the body manufacture GTH. Healthy persons taking 500 mg of Vitamin C daily for two weeks had their GTH levels rise by 50%.

Other substances that may also help the body make GTH include alpha lipoic acid, glutamine, methionine, S adenosyl methionine (SAME), n-acetyl cysteine and whey.

GTH is composed of three amino acids; glycine, glutamic acid and cysteine. Some researchers feel that the best approach may be to present the body with n-acetyl cysteine and allow the body to assemble the glutathione from this precursor. *Taking 600 mg. daily of n-acetyl-cysteine has been shown to increase blood plasma levels of glutathione by 38%.* N-acetyl-cysteine can be purchased from Jo Mar Laboratories 800-538-4545 and from *Natural Health Team* 800-416-2806.

The role of GTH in aging may relate to the ability of GTH to regulate protein synthesis and DNA biosynthesis and cell growth. There is a direct relationship between the life span of a species and it's ability to repair DNA. When DNA is damaged, if GTH or another antioxidant is available the GTH attaches to the damaged area and DNA repair occurs. If no GTH or suitable antioxidant is available the oxygen fixes to the site and the damage is permanent. *When we increase our ability to repair DNA we are slowing the aging process.*

Mutations or damage to DNA strands are linked to cancer. Tobacco, hormones such as estrogen, drugs (legal and illegal), asbestos, coal tar products, benzene, cadmium, uranium, and nickel all can promote DNA damage leading to cancer.

Some observers believe that the well documented health benefits of antioxidants may relate to their ability to elevate the level of glutathione.

Melatonin

Melatonin protects against free radicals in cells and in fat containing membranes. Melatonin also increases the production of Glutathione Peroxidase. This compound is regarded as the premier substance to prevent free radical damage in the human brain.

Melatonin is joined by pycnogenol (pine bark or grape seed extract), bilberry extract, and turmeric (cucurmin) and Vitamin C in their ability to elevate GTH levels.

Cholesterol, when oxidized in the blood, sticks to the lipoprotein(a) at the site of vessel injury and begins the cholesterol plaque problem in the wall of an artery. French researchers have shown that *low levels of GTH in the blood are directly related to increased amounts of oxidized fats in the blood.*

Nearly every cataract is correlated with low levels of GTH in the lens. A traditional Chinese medicine, Ba Wei Wan, is able to raise GTH in the lens. This suggests it could stop or perhaps reverse cataracts. This can be obtained from 1st Chinese Herbs 888-842 2049. The same deficiency of GTH has been linked to age related macular degeneration a common problem in the elderly.

GTH is critical in helping our body detoxify drugs and foreign chemicals. *The ingestion of acetaminophen (Tylenol, AMP) depletes the GTH and cysteine stores in the liver, lungs, and kidneys.*

Animal experiments have shown a rapid fall in GTH level after acetaminophen. Older animals were only able to restore 41% of the level, which existed before acetaminophen was administered. Low levels of GTH in the elderly liver would afford a possible explanation for why elderly persons have great trouble metabolizing drugs. Some young persons taking several days of acetaminophen for an illness have been known to develop acute necrosis of the liver and proceeded to die. They had no history of excessive use of alcohol.

Acetaminophen may be capable of speeding up the aging process. AMP is known to be a powerful generator of free radicals. There are many other pain treatments available, so AMP should be considered as *possibly a dangerous agent that may accelerate aging.* Any treatment that depletes the body of glutathione has to be regarded as dangerous. For an elderly person to take acetaminophen (Tylenol) regularly is a recipe for disaster.

I would suggest reviewing the content of all cold and pain over the counter medicines and consider not purchasing *any formulation containing AMP, as this is in many of those compounds.*

Be sure your multivitamin contains riboflavin (B2), selenium, zinc, and magnesium. All have a role in proper GTH metabolism.

Are there other substances that may help with longevity? Yes.

Melatonin

As discussed in Chapter 7, melatonin is an effective antioxidant protecting the brain, heart, and other organs from free radical injury. This substance also gives a boost to the immune system. By regulating the endocrine system, *melatonin increases the output of growth hormone, which is regarded as the most effective anti-aging compound known.*

Growth Hormone

In an article that appeared in the 1990 New England Journal of Medicine, Dr. Daniel Rudman and his colleagues at The University of Wisconsin released the results of their treatment of 12 men aged 61 to 80 with intramuscular growth hormone. After 6 months, these 12 men had lost 14% of their body fat and gained an average of 8.8% muscle mass. Their bone density increased and their skin became thicker and firmer. Wrinkles disappeared and sexual performance was improved in several. Dr. Rudman concluded that, *"The overall deterioration of the body that comes with growing old is not inevitable. These injections appear able to reverse 10 years of aging with one year of treatment."*

Peter Smith, who was a key person in the development of soil based organisms, has developed a water-based polymer that is able to deliver amino acid nutrient neurotransmitters to the pituitary gland where they stimulate the secretion of physiologic amounts of growth hormone.

The amino acid neurotransmitters include l-arginine, which stimulates HGH output. This also improves male sexual performance, helps burn fat, build muscle, improves thymic function, builds immunity, promotes healing, helps protects the liver, and detoxifies noxious substances.

L-ornithine is twice as potent at releasing HGH as arginine.

L-glutamine Aids in health and growth of muscle tissue as well as releasing HGH.

L-glycine Corrects hyperacidity, aids in construction of RNA and DNA and stabilizes heart and muscle function after heavy exercise.

L-cystine stimulates white blood cell function for disease resistance, needed for skin formation and promotes healing after surgery and burns.

L-taurine assists in lowering blood pressure, lowering cholesterol and triglycerides, and has a calming effect.

L-valine Found in high amounts in muscle tissue.

L-tyrasine Precursor substance for adrenaline and thyroid hormones. Aids in control of depression and anxiety. Suppresses appetite and has antioxidant properties.

GABA (gamma amino butyric acid) helps regulate the anterior pituitary gland where HGH is secreted.

The results of 28,000 studies around the world show that growth hormone often provides:

- Increased muscle mass without exercise

- Loss of fat without dieting

- Improved sexual function

- Reduction of wrinkles

- Regrowth of heart, liver, spleen, and kidneys to a more youthful size

- Increased cardiac output

- Better kidney function

- Lower blood pressure

- Stronger bones

- Faster healing of wounds

- Improved immune function

- More youthful skin

- Higher energy level

- Improved cholesterol level

- Hair regrowth and restoration of hair color

- Improved vision

- Improved sleep and mood elevation

- Improved memory

Note: After several months of growth hormone an individual may experience several changes. At this point he or she will need to decide if the benefits warrant continuation of therapy with GTH.

Too much growth hormone can cause high blood pressure, elevation of blood sugar values, carpal tunnel syndrome and fluid retention.

This natural growth hormone product is aptly named *Young Again*. It is supplied in a one-ounce atomizer and should be taken two sprays three times daily under the tongue. The preferable time to take this is 30 minutes before all three meals. If you must take after a meal, wait two hours before using.

Young Again was first primarily used by world class athletes, but has now been released for use by the general public. This can be obtained from *Natural Health Team* 800-416-2806.

Dihydroepiandosterone (DHEA)

DHEA has been shown to have highly significant reductions in both mortality and deaths from heart disease, when given to patients with heart disease. The mechanism for this striking benefit is not clear but may relate to lowered production of cholesterol and fatty acids.

The steady, severe fall in DHEA with aging may have undesirable health consequences, as there is an associated decrease in hormone levels. *Replacement of one of these hormones (growth hormone) is clearly beneficial.*

Millions of Americans now take DHEA, which is available in health food stores. DHEA is a precursor to the production of testosterone, estrogen, and other sex hormones.

Another important action of DHEA is to counteract stress. When under chronic stress, the level of cortisone remains elevated. This causes increased heart rate, elevated blood pressure, and high amounts of cortisone in brain tissue. When cortisone levels are high, the DHEA levels are low. Even young individuals under stress exhibit very low DHEA.

A consequence of this high cortisone level in the brain is malfunction of the hippocampus, where memories and learning are processed. *As cortisone levels rise there is a fall in DHEA, which results in decreased attention and memory.*

Dr. Samuel Yen at the Universityof San Diego gave 50 mg. of DHEA daily to men and 25 mg. daily to women between the ages of 40 and 70. After three months, 67% of men and 84% of women reported significant improvements in mood, sleep, energy, and ability to cope with stress.

DHEA also appears to restore proper immune function. Elderly persons are known to have decreased function of the immune system, which lowers resistance to infection. DHEA curbs the injurious effects of cortisone, which leads to better immune function. DHEA is also a powerful antioxidant, and enhances the activity of cytokines, which act to mobilize the immune system.

Studies have also shown that DHEA increases the activity of killer lymphocytes and may even help protect against cancer. Because of these many beneficial effects and lack of any clearly adverse effects, consider starting long-term therapy with DHEA beginning at age 40.This therapy needs to be monitored with regular blood tests so the dosage can be appropriately changed as needed.

All men should have a blood PSA and rectal exam before starting DHEA. This needs to be repeated annually as there is a theoretical risk of activating prostate cancer if the DHEA causes testosterone levels to rise.DHEA is available from *Natural Health Team* 800-416-2806.

Fasting

A discussion of longevity would not be complete without including fasting Occasional short term fasting of 2 to 3 days has many proven *physical* benefits to the body.

A study of very old persons disclosed that many had practiced periodic fasting during their lives. *During periods of fasting the body is able to eliminate toxins from the liver and other organs and the metabolic efforts to digest food is eliminated. This is a significant benefit to health.*

The value of short term fasting is so clearly documented that there is even a rough, general "formula" to estimate how much life is extended by periodical short term fasting. Paavo Airola, a noted health care expert, estimated that fasting three days monthly extends life by 5 to 7 years. Of course, this is a rough estimate. However, there is no question that periodic, short term (2 to 3 days) fasting, giving the body a chance to "take a break" and eliminate toxins from organs, is highly beneficial to general health.

Chapter 26

Dementia In The Elderly (Alzheimer's Disease)

The diagnosis of Alzheimer's Disease (A. D.) is difficult to establish. A. D. appears to be a disease of "advanced civilization", as there are more than 4 million persons in the U.S. with the disease. In poorly developed parts of the world, the disease is practically nonexistent. This suggests that there is some agent commonly experienced by our advanced societies that is not a factor in life styles in other parts of the world.

There is no doubt that modern man is exposed to aluminum in a steady, insistent manner. For example, we use antiperspirants that often contain aluminum, along with antacids for heartburn that also may contain aluminum.

There is evidence that aluminum may leach into our food from aluminum cooking utensils and cans as well as from frequent use of aluminum foil to wrap our food. Many cities use alum (aluminum) in water treatment to precipitate metals out of the water. Aluminum compounds are widely used in baking.

What Is The Evidence That Alzheimer's Disease Is Caused By Aluminum?

In the 1970's patients with Alzheimer's Disease were found to have blood levels of aluminum that were 1.4 times greater than normal persons. Subsequent studies determined that the aluminum content in the characteristic brain lesion, nerve "tangles", contained very high levels of aluminum. A later study revealed that aluminum blood levels in patients with dementia were *three to four times higher* than in normal healthy persons. *Hip fracture cases had significantly higher levels of aluminum in bone samples taken from patients with Alzheimer's Disease than in bone samples taken from normal persons with hip fractures.*

A group of 48 patients with Alzheimer's Disease were treated with desferrioxamine injections twice daily for 5 days each week for a period of two years. This drug binds aluminum (chelation) so it is excreted in the urine. There was slower deterioration in these patients when compared to patients who did not receive the injections.

In another study, rabbits were given aluminum injections into brain cells to create Alzheimer's type degeneration. Later half the rabbits were given desferrioxamine and half received nothing. The animals that did not receive the anti-aluminum treatment suffered much more neurone damage than the treated animals.

Why Do Some People Get Alzheimer's Disease While Others Do Not?

Most people are able to excrete the aluminum in urine without difficulty. There is some research evidence that deficiencies of essential fatty acids may cause injury to cell membranes that permits aluminum to enter tissues that are normally safe from aluminum deposits. *Such fatty acid deficiencies are widespread in the US population.*

Good kidney function is needed to be able to eliminate aluminum effectively, which could mean that persons with borderline or diminished kidney function are more likely to encounter trouble with brain deposits of aluminum. This is certainly true for uremic patients.

There is clear evidence that individuals who ingest large quantities of aluminum are at an increased risk. In a study, 23 persons with Alzheimer's disease were compared with 23 similar normal persons. The researchers learned that the persons with Alzheimer's Disease had a high lifetime consumption of pancakes, waffles, biscuits, muffins and other baked goods, which *doubled* their chance of developing Alzheimer's Disease. All these bakery products contain baking powder, which has considerable aluminum used to leaven the product.

Deposits in the Alzheimer's "tangles" are particularly heavy in the olfactory lobe region of the brain. This is where stimuli from smell are processed. This is also where the inhaled aluminum from spray type antiperspirants would appear. Almost certainly, users of spray antiperspirants and deodorants containing aluminum are at increased risk for Alzheimer's Disease. For most persons the use of antiperspirants may be the greatest source of aluminum. Many antacids contain aluminum, as do some cosmetics.

Cookware is another source for aluminum and aluminum pots, pans and utensils as well as cans are leaching aluminum into our food and beverages. Researchers in Australia studied 106 cans containing 52 different beverages and found that non-cola beverages in cans had *five times the aluminum content* as the same drink when packaged in a glass bottle.

What Should Be Done To Prevent The Development Of Alzheimer's Disease And To Help Persons With The Disease?

Stop using products, which contain aluminum. This means our aluminum kitchen utensils need to be replaced with cookware from glass, porcelain or coated in a high-quality nonstick surface like Silver Stone or Baker's Secret. Purchase food and beverage in glass containers instead of aluminum cans and use deodorants that contain no aluminum. Avoid the use of aluminum foil. Wrap foods in cellophane or cardboard instead of aluminum foil. (The cooked food could react chemically with the aluminum in the foil.) Do not purchase antacids containing aluminum. Drink filtered water, as alum is used to purify water. Cease using baking powder in baking and do not buy commercial baking products containing aluminum. This means you will have to avoid most commercially baked pies, cakes or cookies.

It is far more important (and easy) to keep aluminum out of your body than to try to remove it after it has done its damage.

My belief is that attempting to remove aluminum from victims of Alzheimer's Disease with chelation or DNF should slow their deterioration and might possibly arrest further decline. Some might even get better. *Research to uncover which chelating agents remove the most aluminum could be very valuable.*

One patient of Dr. Robert D. Willix was of considerable interest to me. This patient had dementia caused by brain atrophy. She was confused, having delusions and frequently unable to recognize her husband. When she left her home she could not find her way back. Following her first six months infusions of EDTA *she recovered normal mentation with disappearance of all signs of confusion.*

EDTA is known to be a powerful antioxidant as well as removing metals from the body Brain atrophy is regarded as a hopeless situation because large numbers of neurons have been destroyed by some disease process decreasing the size of the brain. Brain cells do not regenerate, so I would not have expected any improvement in this women.. Probably the chelation led to removal of some toxin that interfered with normal brain function. *Clearly her atrophic brain was still capable of normal function.*

Dr. Marcial Veaga has noted disappearance of *schizophrenia* after several months of oral NDF. This mode of therapy which uses atomized chlorella, cilantro and vitamins is capable of bringing about unexpected benefits. Much research is needed to find out more about the reasons for improvement with this therapy. NDF is more effective at removing mercury than intravenous chelation, so it would appear worth trying in Alzheimer's Disease as it does remove aluminium.

Probably two or three months of treatment should give evidence whether improvement will be forthcoming.

Much of the information about the role aluminum plays in causing Alzheimer's Disease was obtained from the September, 2000 issue of *To Your Health* by Dr. John A. McDougall. Several years ago Dr. McDougall was strongly condemned by spokesmen for the aluminum industry when he pointed out the connection between aluminum and Azheimer's Disease on a national radio program. He challenged the aluminum spokesmen to a debate. *No reply was received.*

The connection between aluminum and Alzheimer's Disease perhaps also provides the explanation for a remarkable fact: Alzheimer's Disease is almost never found in undeveloped countries.

Pernicious Anemia And Dementia

Approximately 10% of the U.S. population over age 70 have low or low normal B12 values and metabolic evidence of B 12 deficiency (elevated levels of homocysteine and methylmalonic acid) that return to normal with B 12 therapy. *Therapy of these persons with B 12 may well prevent dementia from developing.*

These 3 tests are used to screen patients for the disease pernicious anemia. *Individuals with high blood levels of homocysteine or methylmalonic acid are 4.5 times more likely to develop A.D. than persons with low levels of homocysteine and methyl malonic acid. The dementia developing in these persons is probably the dementia which is widely recognized to occur in pernicious anemia (PA) and has nothing to do with Alzheimer's Disease.*

In a Norwegian study all patients admitted to a mental hospital bed had B 12 blood levels checked. They found that the percentage of hospitalized mental patients having a low B 12 was thirty times that of similar age non-hospitalized patients. *This percentage of abnormal results would have certainly been much high had methyl malonic and homocysteine been evaluated as these two tests are much more sensitive to the detection of PA than is the B 12 level.*

This information reveals that serious abnormalities in brain function, including dementia caused by PA are very common and are often undiagnosed. Looking for PA in mental institutions can be very rewarding, as hundreds of institutionalized patients have returned to normal following B 12 injections.

The psychiatric symptoms of paranoia, confusion, psychosis, memory loss and personality change that can be seen in PA are impossible to differentiate from the dementia symptoms in Alzheimer's Disease. For this reason we suggest obtaining homocysteine and methyl malonic blood tests on all persons with dementia. It is tragic to consign an individual to a nursing home or mental facility when they have a treatable disease. Also, underactive thyroid function, normal pressure hydrocephalus, brain tumor and severe depression need to be excluded in demented persons.

Some people suspected of having Alzheimer's Disease actually have Pernicious Anemia. Treating these persons with B 12 prevents them from developing permanent dementia.

Galantamine

Galantamine is a natural flower extract obtained from snowdrop, daffodil, and spider lily. This substance blocks the action of cholinesterase but this benefit does not wear off, which is the problem with Cognex.

Galantamine also stimulates acetylcholine receptors for an extended period of time. In A.D. patients, the acetylcholine receptors wear out and the brain becomes unable to transport acetylcholine from one cell to another. When these acetylcholine receptors are healthy, they are believed to be important in preventing the formation of amyloid plaques in the brain, a change frequently seen in A.D.

Researchers in New Zealand have shown that 24 mg daily of galantamine for 3 to 6 months was followed by improved cognition and activities of daily living, compared to placebo controls in patients with A.D. After 12 months, these patients taking galantamine maintained their improved cognitive and functional ability.

Research on 3000 A.D. patients in Belgium revealed that galantamine patients maintained their cognition, while other control test patients deteriorated over a 12 month follow up.

Galantamine has side effects of nausea, vomiting and diarrhea in some patients, which can be overcome by using smaller initial doses.

Parkinson's Disease, multiple sclerosis, and myasthenia gravis might also be helped by galantamine treatment.

Galantamine can be obtained from Life Enhancement Products, Inc. Phone 800-543 3873

Reversal Of "Normal" Brain Aging With Vinpocetine

Elderly individuals often have trouble remembering names, tell the same story twice without realizing it, miss appointments, have memory lapses, and forget words and names. The brain requires a disproportionately large portion of the heart's cardiac output for its size. *Because of this, the brain is very sensitive to impaired brain circulation.* The natural substance vinpocetine has three beneficial qualities to improve brain function:

It causes a *selective* increase in the quantity of blood flowing to the brain.

Blood is also directed in increased quantity to any area of the brain that has been injured, such as by a stroke. This speeds up healing. By inhibiting the tendency of platelets to clump blood, oxygenation into the brain is improved.

Vinpocetine seems to improve brain metabolism by increasing the brain's utilization of oxygen. This is associated with an improved ability to withstand a deficit of oxygen. such as would appear after a stroke. By regulating phosphodiesterase and adenyl cyclase, vincopetine increases brain ATP which is the primary source of energy for brain function.

This increase in brain oxygen improves cognitive functions of the brain. Worldwide trials are showing improvement in memory, concentration, speech, communication, dizziness, and co-ordination after vincopetine usage. Combination of vinpocetine with other brain active nutrients gingko, acetyl-l-carnitine, phosphatidylserine and bacopa monniera could increase the overall beneficial effect.

Ginko increases circulation to the brain and is an anti-oxidant.

Acetyl-l-carnitine prevents brain cell death and protects nerve cells from aging or disease. This substance easily crosses into brain tissue where it stimulates mitochondria, the energy factory for brain cells and leads to greater alertness, improved learning, and better memory.

Phosphatidylserine (PS) is an essential fatty acid that allows brain cells to better absorb nutrients. It has been shown to improve memory and learning in the most severe cases.

Bacopa monniera is a natural botanical substance that improves recall and reaction time. This may act as an antioxidant and as a chelator of heavy metals.

This formulation is called MEMORACTIV and is available from Center for Natural Medicine Dispensary, Portland, Oregon. Ph: 888-305-4288.

Chapter 27

Eye Diseases

Cataracts

Cataracts are a degenerative process in the lens that leads to the inability to see through the lens, which becomes opaque. The standard treatment for this condition is surgical removal of the lens and implantation of a new lens. 4 million people in the U.S.A. have cataracts and 400,000 are blind from this condition. When the glutathione level in the lens falls a cataract appears.

New advances in medicine have brought about the ability to dissolve the opacities in the lens and restore normal vision. An ancient Chinese herbal remedy (Ba Wei Wan or Hachimijiogan) used to restore the function to degenerating organs, was tested by Japanese researchers. They recently discovered that this ancient substance raised HDL (good) and lowered LDL (bad) cholesterol. *This herb also raised the glutathione level in the lens. This strongly suggests that this herbal compound might dissolve cataracts.*

Ba Wei Wan can be obtained from 1st Chinese Herbs 888-8422049.They also sell a herbal product called Liu Wei Di Huang Wan, which is an updated version of Ba Wei Wan.

In 1974 Dr. Gary Price Todd, an opthalmologist, took care of a patient with blindness in both eyes from cataracts .He operated on one eye and prescribed Vitamin E, zinc, and other nutrients. When the patient returned for the second cataract operation, her vision had improved to 20/25 and the surgery was cancelled. *Antioxidants had dissolved the opacity in the lens.*

Vitamin C is important in the prevention of cataracts. *A healthy lens has the highest concentration of Vitamin C in the body, while a lens burdened by a cataract has very little.* In a study of 121,700 nurses, those who took Vitamin C for ten years or more *had far fewer cataracts than those who did not take Vitamin C.*

Immunocal

(See CHAPTER 2) Immunocal is a preparation of milk-serum-proteins that builds cellular glutathione. A patient named Henry Cheang was known to have early stage full lens cataracts. He began immunocal therapy and 4 months later his cataracts were gone. This should not be considered surprising, because the lens is known to be lacking glutathione when a cataract develops.

St. Lucia Drops

These drops are prepared from the herb atel cugel.

Dr. Victor Marcial-Vega of Health Horizons Rejuvenation Clinic, Coral Gables, Fl. (www.healthhorizonsinc.com) claims that St.Lucia drops eliminate cataracts, eye infections, glaucoma, retinitis and ptergium. One drop is applied to the eye at bedtime nightly. Results appear in two weeks.

Dr. Marcial-Vega relates that dissolution of the cataracts will be followed by reappearance of the cataracts if life style changes are not accomplished. This means that the conditions that caused the cataracts to appear (cigarettes, alcohol, poor diet, lack of vitamins and antioxidants) need to be changed to get permanent visual improvement. This product can be obtained from Health Horizons,305 442- 1233 or 800 771-0255 and from our *Natural Health Team* 800-416-2806.

Melatonin

Melatonin production by the pineal gland has nearly ceased at age 60.

In an experiment on newborn rats using a drug that interfered with glutathione synthesis, cataracts were produced. Half the rats were given melatonin and only 6.2% of these rats developed cataracts, whereas all the untreated rats had cataracts. This gives another potential reason for taking melatonin daily.

The common belief that sunlight (UV ultraviolet) causes cataracts may be incorrect. Cataracts are less common in the tropics where sunlight is plentiful. UV light may actually protect against cataract development.

Macular Degeneration

Macular degeneration has become one of the leading causes of blindness in persons over 55. Heredity and smoking are important risk factors for macular degeneration.

The back of the eye contains a critical area called the macula where visual images are focused. A vast network of nerve fibers is present in this region that transmit visual signals to the brain. These signals enable us to read fine print and pick out a face in a crowd. Studies have suggested that free radical damage to the macula may be responsible for age related macular degeneration (ARMD). Patients with ARMD have low blood levels of glutathione.

Past research has shown that several supplements can halt ARMD. These include Vitamin E, Vitamin C, Selenium, Ginko biloba and huckleberry. Four atoms of selenium are needed to build an atom of glutathione peroxidase, a crucial enzyme. Patients deficient in selenium have lower glutathione activity and adding 200 mg of selenium rich yeast to the diet daily raises the activity of glutathione.

Macular degeneration can be prevented by ingestion of carotenoids (spinach, tomatoes, green vegetables, grapes, yellow and green onions, and green tea.) Zinc taken in 30 mg daily halts visual loss in ARMD.

Taurine is critical for nerve impulse formation. The dose is 500 to 600 mg daily. Dr. Robert Atkins reports that vision improves after one injection of intravenous taurine.

Bilberry was found to lead to a significant improvement in night vision by British pilots in WW 2. Bilberry has antioxidant properties and improves blood flow to the eyes. The dose is 60 mg daily of standardized extract

Ginko biloba is also an antioxidant, which helps circulation to small blood vessels. The dose is 60 to 160 mg daily of standardized extract. Avoid regular use of aspirin, which appears to be a possible risk factor for ARMD when taken on a regular basis.

Retinitis Pigmentosa

This condition is associated with pigmentation of the retina. When this pigment deposit involves the macula, visual loss occurs.

New Ideas For Treating Age Related Macular Degeneration And Retinitis Pigmentosa

Three Doctors of Optometry at the University of Indiana Medical School (Dr. Leland Michael, Dr. Ralph Zehner and Dr. Merril Allen) have achieved wonderful results in therapy of these two disorders. The basic therapy for both is a specific nutritional formulation for each disease:

Beta-Carotene	40,000 units
Vitamin E(natural)	400 I.U.
Vitamin C	1500 mg
Citrus Bioflavinoid Complex	250 mg.

Quercetin	100 mg.
Bilberry Extract	10 mg
Rutin	100 mg
Zinc	100 mg
Selenium	100 mg
Taurine	200mg
N-acetylcysteine	200 mg
L-glutathione	10 mg
Vitamin B	250 mg

Retinitis Pigmentosa patients receive a multi mineral and vitamin formula with 750 mg of taurine, 300 mg. of bilberry and 50 mg. of zinc.

46 patients with ARMD took the supplement for two years. Visual deterioration would normally be expected in these patients. *Their vision improved instead of deteriorating.*

Each patient also received micro current electricity using 200 microamperes at 10 cycles per second (Hz). One electrode is placed in the patient's wet hand and the other gently placed on a closed wet eye. Each eye is stimulated for 5 minutes using 2.5 minutes for the upper and the same time for the lower lid. Using the micro TENS several times daily seemed to increase the benefit.

The micro current seemed to improve blood flow to the retina and also permitted *regeneration of the retina.* One patient's retina had been surgically removed. After nine months of therapy the *retina regenerated and vision improved to 20/40. Another 80 year old patient with ARMD regained normal vision after 12 years of treatment.*

Some patients who had been told to learn Braille are now driving cars. The micro current Tens units cost about $150. Isn't it fascinating that the micro current used in the orthopedic patches and the micro current used in the eye both appear to heal with lower than standard TENS UNIT currents?

Micro Tens units can be purchased from Altoona Medical Supply 800-4428367

Lasik Surgery For Myopia

Lasik surgery (laser-assisted in-situ Keratomilusis) uses lasers to reshape the cornea so glasses or no longer needed. This procedure has become the latest fad in cosmetic surgery. Two million persons will have this operation this year. The surgery has become a $3 to $5 billion industry. Consider avoiding this procedure because the long-term consequences are yet to be fully known. As in any surgery complications may occur. There is a great variation in the skills of the physicians performing this procedure. Many doctors have learned how to do this procedure operating on pig eyes at a weekend seminar.

Only 5% of cases are estimated to have complications from this surgery. Some unfortunate people have worse permanent vision after the operation.

One of the common problems post operatively is seeing starbursts, glare, halos or "ghosting" around lights at night. One study found this in 12% of Lasik patients one year after the surgery. *Many individuals are unable to drive at night because of this problem.*

Other problems include incomplete healing, dry eyes and a loss of visual contrast. Incomplete healing can lead to infections and permanent scarring. All persons undergoing this procedure will have dry eyes for a few weeks. Usually this is temporary and responds to eye drops. In some cases, however, the nerves are severed when the cornea is cut and this results in loss of sensation and a permanent inability to produce adequate tears. *Some people have to use eye drops every five minutes while awake and every hour during the night.*

The loss of contrast can be even more serious. Three years ago reports began to appear from Great Britain and elsewhere that the loss of contrast was so severe that between 30% and 60% of Lasik patients were unable to pass sensitivity test for night driving. This loss of contrast sensitivity makes it difficult to pick out dark object against a light background or light objects against a dark background.

Some persons have noted double vision, triple vision, permanent dry eyes and inability to drive at night. When successful this operation often improves distant vision at the expense of near vision.

The lens and the macula continue to change as we age. *Successful Lasik surgery today provides no guarantee that you might not need glasses again 10 or 15 years later.* Some leading opthamologists have expressed concern that the procedure permanently ruins the cornea so *visual correction later may not be possible.*

Recently, the FDA suggested only those persons willing to take a risk should have Lasik surgery. I suggest you think very carefully before you proceed with Lasik surgery.

Eye Blend For Hyperopia (Farsighted Vision) And Eye Infections

EYE BLEND contains a proprietary blend of essential oils from plants and herbs that were initially used to clear eye infections. One of the oils is jasmine.

After usage, patients returned saying that they were no longer farsighted and had been able to give up using glasses. Dr. Marcial-Vega believes that this herbal blend may be opening up the drainage canals for the eye that have become partially occluded over many years.

One drop is applied to the upper and lower eyelid of each eye at bedtime. Generally a few days are needed for the vision to return to normal. The blend is fat- soluble. Eye infections respond promptly.

EYE BLEND is available from Health Horizons 305 442- 1233 or 1800 771-0255 and from our *Natural Health Team* 800-416-2806.

Chapter 28

Resistant Bacteria, Candida (Yeast), And Viruses

The head of the Central Public Health Laboratory in London recently reported that a new drug resistant strain of salmonella typhimurium (ST) had infected 4,000 people in Great Britain. These bacteria resist 98.8% of the available antibiotics. Fortunately, this strain was not very virulent but this drug resistance could and does spread to other bacteria.

Several years ago tuberculosis was widely believed to be a defeated disease. Last year the highest number of deaths in history from tuberculosis occurred (3,000,000). This disease afflicts alcoholics, drug addicts, and HIV patients and is more common where poverty, overcrowding and poor nutrition are problems.

Because many patients with tuberculosis are unable to keep up the treatment, the prescribed course of antibiotics is often not completed (6 months to 2 years may be needed). The incomplete treatment gives the tuberculosis bacteria a greater chance to become resistant to the drugs that were being given.

When drug resistance for tuberculosis appears, it engenders new problems. The antibiotic drugs for drug resistant tuberculosis are often very toxic, which encourages non - compliance. They are also very expensive. The complete course of treatment may cost $250,000 per person. Naturally, not many governments can afford to treat these patients.

What Can Be Done?

New approaches are needed. Malaria has become a very serious global problem. In a recent year between 300 million and 500 million cases of malaria occurred and nearly 3,000,000 persons died. Drug resistant strains are common. The best current treatment may be a Chinese herb called Qing hao, which has been used effectively for decades in China.

E. coli is the most prevalent bacteria in the gastrointestinal tract. A mutant form of E.coli appeared in the U.S. in contaminated meat served at a Seattle fast food chain. 50 persons developed internal bleeding and 4 small children died.

Some of the reason for this problem may lie in over prescription of antibiotics by physicians. However, another cause is giving antibiotics to animals so they grow faster and bigger. *Healthy chicken and cattle are routinely fed antibiotics. The epidemic of salmonella in England and the E. coli epidemic at a Seattle fast food restaurant were both linked to giving livestock antibiotics.*

I recommend an excellent special report from *Alternatives*: *Defend Yourself From The New Mutant Bacteria* published by Mountain Home Publishing of Potomac, Md.

Recently the Union of Concerned Scientists released a study showing that while the overuse and abuse of antibiotics by medical doctors is a key factor in the bacterial resistance problem, *the use of anti-microbials in agriculture may play an even more significant role.*

This report said "Tetracycline, penicillin, erthromycin and other antimicrobials that are important in human use are used extensively in the absence of disease for nontherapeutic purposes in today's livestock production. Cattle, swine, and poultry are routinely given antimicrobials throughout much of their lives. "

Why is this done? *Antibiotics are an inexpensive way to get animals "fatted for market" earlier than normal.*

Livestock producers in the U.S. are estimated to use 24.6 million pounds of antibiotics for non-therapeutic (fattening) purposes annually. Obviously many more millions of pounds of antibiotics are used to care for sick animals. You are absorbing some of those antibiotics when you eat these products. The quantity of antibiotics used by agriculture dwarf the 3 million pounds used to treat disease in humans. This means that 8 times more antibiotics are used to fatten animals than are used to treat human diseases.

This abuse has contributed significantly to the development of bacterial resistance. Currently 10.5 million pounds of antibiotics are used to fatten poultry, 10.3 million pounds are used to fatten swine and 3.7 million pounds are used to fatten cattle. *Non- therapeutic livestock use amounts to 70% of total production of antibiotics.* The pharmaceutical industry has a very lucrative business here. Accurate figures are hard to come by, as the industry admits only 40% of total antibiotic production is going to agriculture, which seems far too low.

In the January/February issue of *FDA Consumer* the headline story, *"Antibiotic Resistance Down On The Chicken Farm"*, details information about actions taken by the Center for Veterinary Medicine (CVM) to address this problem. The CVM proposed that permission to sell Baytril (enrofloxin), a Bayer product, for use in chickens and turkeys be withdrawn. Enrofloxin is a quinilone antibiotic, which is a type of antibiotic widely used to treat human diseases. The poultry industry has been using the quinilone antibiotics to control the resistant mutant form of e.coli that can kill humans.

The *FDA Consumer* relates that the size of flocks precludes testing and treating an individual chicken, so an ill bird causes the whole flock to receive antibiotics in their water. This has cured the e.coli in the poultry, but a worse problem has developed.

Campylobacter has now built up resistance to quinilones. Since campylobacter has become the most common cause of diarrhoeal illness in the U.S. today, we now face the frightening prospect that many of the 2,000,000 annual cases of campylobacter seen in the U.S. will be resistant to the quinilone type of antibiotic. Campylobacter infections can kill persons with weakened immune systems and campylobacter can be found in chickens sold in markets.

When antibiotics are used they kill all gastrointestinal bacteria that are sensitive to the antibiotic used. This leaves more harmful bacteria that were in small numbers a chance to greatly multiply. It also gives candida yeast a great opening to multiply as well, because conventional antibiotics have no effect on candida. Many women fear taking an antibiotic because they know they will get a yeast infection in their vagina. Currently, it is believed that a high percentage of chickens sold are contaminated with salmonella or campylobacter bacteria.

How Can This Threat Be Resolved?

Programs to try to explain to farmers why the use of antibiotics is creating a worse problem than having slightly smaller and slightly slower growing animals could be beneficial. In a recent year 35.2% of chicken broilers tested positive for salmonella. 12% of pork and 1.8% of beef were also positive for salmonella. If the general public becomes afraid to buy meat and chickens, it will get the farmers' attention.

Another simple solution will certainly help. *Placing beneficial forms of bacteria and yeast in animal food instead of antibiotics could work.*

In an experiment, a friendly yeast (saccharymyces boulardii) was added to the feed of one half a group of chickens. All the chickens were then given salmonella by mouth. *The salmonella were only able to establish growth in 5% of the chickens getting yeast (probiotic) whereas they were able to establish growth in 70% of the chickens not given yeast.*

Drug Resistant Enterocci

In the past, enterococci were not a common bacterial problem and when seen, they responded well to vancomycin therapy. Enterococci are normal inhabitants of our intestinal tract, but are much less frequent than E. coli.

In 1988, some strains of enterococci began to appear in a New York City Hospital *that were resistant to vancomycin (VRE)*. By October 1991, 38 hospitals had discovered vancomycin resistant enterococci in cultures from their patients. 98 of 100 patients with VRE had contacted these bacteria in the hospital. This problem spread over the whole nation. The Center for Disease Control reported a 20 fold increase in VRE between Jan, 1,1989 and March 31,1993. Now, VRE is in nearly every country in the world.

The pattern in all nations was the same:

- Nearly all VRE was acquired in hospitals.

- 50% of VRE were found in intensive care units.

- Patients who had been previously treated with vancomycin were at higher risk to get VRE.

- Patients with an underlying serious illness, suppressed immune system or those who had undergone abdominal surgery (pre op antibiotics are routine and may be a bad idea) were at increased risk of VRE.

If VRE enters the bloodstream, there is 100% fatal outcome.

Enterococci are normal inhabitants of the gastrointestinal tract and the vagina. The VRE are easily passed from patient to patient or from hospital personnel to patient, despite careful washing and steady changes of gloves.

There are new antibiotics close to public release that affect many bacteria, but there is no evidence that these will kill VRE. If they do kill VRE how long will it take the enterococci to develop resistance to the new antibiotics?

There is valid concern that bacterial resistance seen in enterococci will start appearing in other similar bacteria.

Can the individual obtain any protection against a possible VRE infection when he enters the hospital? Yes.

There is a wonderful natural antibacterial substance made from grapefruit seed extract. Has it been tried on VRE? Fortunately, yes.

The patient was an elderly lady who received a broad- spectrum antibiotic for pneumonia. Urine culture and a rectal swab grew VRE.

With the patient's approval, she was given a natural treatment from Bio/Chem Research called Capsules Plus which contains 100 mg of grapefruit seed extract, 200 mg of aternisia annua, and 200 mg of Echinacea angusifolia. After three capsules daily, the urine and rectal cultures returned to normal on the 5th day and she was permitted to return to her nursing home.

If no one had known about Capsules Plus, she might have needed to remain in hospital for the remainder of her life, as it is difficult to place patients with a serious infectious problem (VRE) into a nursing home.

Two other patients with VRE at the same hospital have been treated successfully in the same manner.

The ingredients in Capsules Plus also are formulated in a liquid form, (Nutribiotic Liquid Concentrate NLC), that can be used by travelers to purify suspect drinking water and to treat "traveler's diarrhea".

Three to five drops of NLC will purify a glass of water and fifteen to thirty drops will purify a gallon of water. Ten to fifteen drops will stop diarrhea. This might need to be repeated several times.

Nutribiotic (NLC) can be purchased in many health food stores.

It could be a wise precaution to have a health care professional order Capsules Plus for you from Bio/Chem Research 800 225 4345. Having this therapy available to treat a drug-resistant bacterial infection could be life saving, as few hospitals stock this therapy.

Candida Infections

Vaginal candida infections (yeast monilial organisms) can receive 5 natural treatments:

Douche with plain natural yogurt. This will help reestablish healthy flora in the vagina, with clearing of symptoms.

Place a gelatin capsule filled with boric acid in the vagina daily for two weeks. This can be found in a pharmacy. The cure rate is 90% with no side effects.

Douche twice daily with a solution of one part iodine to 100 parts of water. This appears to be a 100% cure.

If the candida appear to have spread throughout the body, get fresh organic garlic from a health food store or supermarket. Take four or five large cloves each day. You may notice a large bowel movement resembling spaghetti, which is the yeast colonies being eliminated. Cut down to one clove daily after two weeks and eat unflavored yogurt daily to reestablish healthy bacteria in your gut.

Take one caspsule of Culturelle daily for one month. This will restore healthy bacteria into the intestinal tract. (See Chapter 17 Gastrointestinal Diseases for information about Culterelle).

Viruses

Dr. Madeleine Mumcuoglu of Israel has invented a wonderful treatment for viral infections. This is an extract of elderberries called Sambucol. When used during the Southern Israeli flu epidemic of 1992, those taking Sambucol were improved in 2 days, while untreated persons only had 16% feeling better in two days. Most patients needed one week to recover.

Why viral vaccines have not been very effective:

If not all the virus particles in the vaccine have been inactivated, the person injected will become infected or get a serious reaction to the injection. Sometimes the immunization does not take and the individual has no protection.

Since a vaccine is specific for only one virus and there are hundreds of viruses that cause cold like symptoms, you are only protected for one of many viruses.

The beauty of Sambucol is that it appears to bind with viruses *before they penetrate the cell wall.* Users of this product claim that if used at the first sign of flu the problem disappears in 24 to 48 hours.

Some viral infections cause serious morbidity, infectious mono, Burkitt's lymphoma, polio, dengue, influenza, measles, mumps, chicken pox, herpes, HIV, meningitis, hepatitis A, B, C, and other types, myocarditis, yellow fever, and hemorrhagic fevers (Lassa, Ebola). Would taking Sambucol in the first 24 to 48 hours stop viral entry into the cell and abort these illnesses?

No one knows, but the potential benefit is so great that having SAMBUCOL available might be life saving. Sambucol has been shown to be effective in defeating a wide variety of viruses. Some individuals stay on Sambucol permanently because they are convinced that flare- ups of herpes progenitalis are prevented.

Consider keeping some SAMBUCOL in your home. The shelf life is 2 years.

We face new dangers of rapid spread of infections because of world wide air travel. This travel permits the spread of serious infections by those who are only incubating an infection or have an undiagnosed illness (influenza, tuberculosis).

Air travel exposes us all to re-circulated air, which is less expensive for the airlines than continuous warming of freezing air brought in from outside the plane. In the same manner, our buildings are now air tight and energy efficient, but cause us to breath re-circulated air, which is more hazardous re infectious disease than fresh air.

Sambucol can be purchased from Mountain Home Nutritionals 800-888 1415 and our *Natural Health Team* 800-416-2806.

Colloidal Silver

Silver has been used to treat infections for many years and was the preferred treatment before the advent of antibiotics. Surgeons have had great success with the topical application of silver solutions to infected burns. The bacteria do not become resistant to the silver solution and *all bacteria, parasite and fungi are responsive to silver therapy.*

Dr. Marchial-Vega has had considerable clinical experience with a colloidal silver preparation that contains between 20 and 25 parts of silver per million parts of water. This preparation has proven effective in patients with HIV in quickly resolving pneumonias due to pnuemocystitis, streptococcal, staphylococcal, klebsiella and fungal infections. In the hospital, the therapy is administered by a special nebulizer as well as orally.

Dr. Vega is confident that this treatment would be effective in treating anthrax infections. It also cures streptococcal throat infection.

The oral dosage is ½ teaspoon three times daily. The preparation is available from Health Horizons 305 442-1233 or 800 771-0255 or from our *Natural Health Team* 800-416-2806.

Chapter 29

Are Immunizations Safe?

To answer this question, a review of the history of immunizations can be valuable. Cowpox vaccine was believed able to immunize people against smallpox. At the time this vaccine was introduced, there was already a decline in the number of cases of smallpox. After widespread use of smallpox vaccine became established in England, a smallpox epidemic broke out that killed 22,081 persons. The smallpox epidemics seemed to get worse each year the vaccine was used. In 1872 44,480 people died.

Japan began compulsory vaccination in 1872. In 1892 there were 165,774 cases of smallpox with 29,979 deaths. Vaccination was compulsory for all servicemen in World War 1. The Boston Herald reported that 47 soldiers died of the vaccination in one month. Military hospitals were full with casualties of the vaccine. Germany instituted compulsory vaccination in 1939. The diphtheria rate rose to 150,000 cases, which might have been coincidental but the neighboring country Norway which did not vaccinate had only 50 cases of diphtheria the same year.

A physician from Indiana, Dr. W. B. Clarke, made an astute observation. He noticed that cancer was practically unknown until vaccination was introduced. He had to care for 200 patients with cancer and *he had never seen a case in an unvaccinated person. Possibly the process of vaccination has an adverse effect on our immune system.*

In the March 4, 1977 issue of *Science,* Jonas and Darrell Salk warn, "Live virus vaccines against influenza or poliomyelitis *may in each instance produce the disease it intended to prevent. The live virus against measles and mumps may produce such side effects as encephalitis (brain damage)* ".

The swine flu vaccine was administered to the American public even though there had never been a case of swine flu identified in a human. Within a few months of use of this vaccine, many cases of nerve injury began to become reported. Claims amounting to $1.3 billion were filed for injury from the vaccine.

In 1986 150 lawsuits were filed against the manufacturers of DPT (Diphtheria, Pertussis, Tetanus) vaccine seeking 1.5 billion in damages.

An article in the Washington Post on January 26, 1988, mentioned that all cases of polio since 1979 had been caused by the polio vaccine with no known cases of polio from a wild strain since 1979. This might have created a perfect situation to discontinue the vaccine, but the vaccine is still used.

Mass vaccination programs have nearly eradicated the childhood infectious diseases from the U.S. However, at the same time there has been a simultaneous increase in the number of children diagnosed with serious autoimmune illnesses. Some of the autoimmune disorders probably have a genetic component, but they may well have been precipitated by an environmental insult like having foreign protein particles, mercury, aluminum, formaldehyde, and other toxic materials injected into the vascular system in the form of immunizations.

In 1999, rotovirus vaccine was recommended by the Centers for Disease Control for all infants. When this vaccine program was instituted several infants died and many had life endangering bowel obstructions. Obviously, there was no evidence that this vaccine would cause such serious problems before the vaccine was released for usage.

The pertussis (whooping cough) vaccine has been responsible for 70% of the claims in the Vaccine Injury Program and Compensation program. This vaccine, which contained whole killed bacteria, caused the same serious neurologic problems seen with pertussis, including encephalitis and permanent brain damage.

A large study from Australia showed that the risk of developing encephalitis from the pertussis vaccine was 5 times greater than from encephalitis after contacting pertussis.

Naturally acquired immunity by illness evolves by spread of a virus from the respiratory tract to the liver, thymus, spleen, and bone marrow. When symptoms begin, the entire immune response has been mobilized to repel the invading virus. This complex immune system response confers life long immunity against the invading virus and prepares the child to respond promptly to an infection by the same virus in the future.

Vaccination, in contrast, results in the persisting of live virus or other foreign antigens within the cells of the body, a situation that may provoke autoimmune reactions as the body attempts to destroy its own infected cells. There is no surprise that autoimmune diseases have risen sharply in this era of universal vaccination.

Dr. John Classen has published 29 articles on vaccine-induced diabetes. At least 8 of 10 children with Type 1 (insulin needing) diabetes have this disease as a result of vaccination. These children have avoided measles, mumps, and whooping cough, *but they have received something far worse: an illness that shortens life by 15 to 20 years and results in a life requiring constant medical care.*

Dr. Classen has shown in Finland, the introduction of hemophilus type b vaccine caused three times as many cases of type 1 diabetes as the number of deaths and brain damage from hemophilus influenza type b it prevented.

In New Zealand the incidence of Type 1 diabetes in children rose by 61% after an aggressive vaccination program against hepatitis B. This same program has been started in the U.S.A. and we can now look forward to many cases of Type 1 diabetes in children. Similar rises of diabetes Type 1 have been seen in England, Italy, Sweden, and Denmark after immunization against Hepatitis B.

In the past 10 years, the number of autistic children has risen between 200 and 500 per cent in every state in the U.S. This sharp increase in autism followed the introduction of MMR vaccine in 1975.

Representative Dan Burton's healthy grandson was given injections for 9 diseases in one day. These injections were followed by autism.

These vaccines contain a preservative of mercury called thimerosal. The boy received 41 times the amount of mercury, which is capable of body harm. Mercury is a neurotoxin that can injure the brain and nervous system. And, tragically, it did.

The number of compulsory vaccine injections has increased from 10 to 36 in the last 25 years. During this period, there has been a simultaneous increase in the number of children suffering learning disabilities and attention deficit disorder. Many of these childhood disabilities are related to intrauterine cerebral damage from maternal cocaine use, but possibly vaccines cause many others.

Another intriguing possible vaccine disability is that a dramatic increase in autoimmune diseases (insulin dependent diabetes mellitus, asthma, multiple sclerosis, lupus, Crohn's Disease, and chronic fatigue syndrome) has occurred which some observers feel is due to trivalent vaccine (Measles, Mumps, and Rubella).

Dr. Len Horowitz (Dentist with a Masters degree from Harvard in Public Health) was an investigator for a dental organization. He was called in to investigate the problem of the Florida dentist who had 29 patients with HIV in his practice.

In the course of unraveling this tragic problem, Dr. Horowitz became very involved in the study of the origin of the HIV infections. His research led to the publication of a book titled, Emerging Viruses: HIV, Ebola, and Vaccines.

Dr. Horowitz became aware that the *animal vaccine pool had become seriously contaminated* so that any vaccine taken has the potential to create a serious health problem. This information is documented in detail in his book, which is available from Tetrahedron Incorporated. Phone 800-336-9266.

Children are now receiving Hepatitis B vaccine at age 18 months. Hepatitis B is a blood borne viral illness that is also transmitted sexually. The vaccine appears to dissipate after about 7 years, so these children may receive three injections of this viral substance before they reach an age where they may become sexually active. This might not seem too horrible if the vaccine were safe but 1% of these vaccinated children develop a serious disabling illness after receiving this vaccine.

I cannot forget Dr. W.B.Clarke's statement *"Cancer was practically unknown until compulsory vaccination with cowpox vaccine began to be introduced. I have had to deal with two hundred cases of cancer, and I never saw a case of cancer in an unvaccinated person"*. This important observation demands an explanation and one now appears forthcoming. *All vaccines given over a short period of time to an immature immune system deplete the thymus gland (the primary gland involved in immune reactions) of irreplaceable immature immune cells.*

Each of these cells could have multiplied and developed an army of valuable cells to combat an infection. When these immune cells have been used up permanent immunity may not appear. The Arthur Research Foundation in Tucson, Az. estimates that *up to 60% of our immune system may be exhausted by multiple mass vaccines(36 are now required for children). Only 10% of immune cells are permanently lost when a child is permitted to develop natural immunity from disease.* There needs to be grave concern about these immune system injuring vaccinations!

Compelling evidence is available that the development of the immune system after contracting the usual childhood diseases matures and renders it capable to fight infection in the future.

The use of multiple vaccines, which prevents natural immunity, promotes the development of allergies and asthma. *A New Zealand study disclosed that 23% of vaccinated children develop asthma compared to zero in unvaccinated children.*

Cancer was a very rare illness in the 1890's. This evidence about immune system injury from vaccination affords a plausible explanation for Dr. Clarke's finding that *only vaccinated individuals got cancer.* Some radical adverse change in health occurred in the early 1900's to permit cancer to explode and vaccinating may be the reason.

Vaccines are an *unnatural* phenomena. My guess is that if enough persons said no to immunizations there would be a striking improvement in general health with nature back in the immunizing business instead of man. Having a child vaccinated should be a choice not a requirement. Medical and religious exemptions are permitted by most states.

If you are forced to immunize your children obtain a notarized statement from the director of the facility that they will accept full financial responsibility for any adverse reaction from the vaccine. Since there is at least a 2% risk of a serious reaction from childhood vaccines they will probably be smart enough to permit your child to escape a dangerous procedure.

Seek more information from the Internet site of National Vaccine Information Center if you have questions. Their website is http://www.909shot,com .

Dr. James R. Shannon, former director of the National Institute of Health, declared that " *The only safe vaccine is one that is never used*".

Chapter 30

Men's Health Issues

Prostatitis

Approximately 50% of men have a problem with prostatitis at some time during their lives. Only 5% of these cases can be clearly blamed on bacterial infections.

Bacterial prostatitis is an uncommon but occasionally serious infection often needing hospitalization. The patient is usually in the 20 to 40 age bracket and frequently has high fever. The patient usually has pain with voiding, frequent urinating, difficulty emptying the bladder, and may note pain in the rectal area, above the bladder, or in the flanks. There is usually severe pain with pressure over the prostate gland.

This illness often responds to the quinolone or trimetaprim sulfametoxazole antibiotics which may need to be continued for 4 weeks.

Chronic prostatitis causes frequent urination, discomfort during urination and mild pain in the prostate area. Cultures obtained by expressing fluid from the prostate gland do not grow bacteria.

Treatment is not always satisfactory. A course of prostate gland massages may be tried or a long course of antibiotics can also be tried. If the symptoms clear, it is difficult to be sure whether the antibiotics helped or if the problem spontaneously healed.

Benign Prostatic Hypertophy

This is invariably a disease of men over the age of 50. The disease is clearly related to testosterone, as it is never seen in castrated males.

An enzyme 5-alpha-reductase converts testosterone to dihydro-testosterone, which is far more active than testosterone in binding to sites in prostate cells that stimulates cell growth. Saw palmetto and Proscar inhibit 5-alpha-reductase.

Recent research suggests that estrogen may play a role in prostate enlargement. Blocking the estrogen dominance of males with natural progesterone (Wild Yam Cream) might prove beneficial. Estrogen dominance will be studied in more detail in Chapter 31, Women's Health Issues.

The symptoms produced by an enlarging prostate gland are occasionally surprisingly few, even in very large glands. Usually there is some decrease in the force of the urinary stream, difficulty initiating urination, and incomplete bladder emptying .The man who is not emptying his bladder completely will urinate and then be able to urinate a considerable amount of urine again in 15 or 20 minutes. In the later stages, urine dribbles out instead of flowing and finally straining to empty the bladder fails to accomplish the passage of any urine (urinary retention which requires catheter drainage of the bladder).

About ten per cent of men will need to have the enlarged prostate gland cored out or removed surgically by the time they reach 80.

The only natural therapy that I know of which decreases the size of the prostate gland is one case treated with SBO. Sterinol (see Chapter 3) has been effective in relieving the symptoms of an enlarged prostate.

Saw Palmetto helps many males with enlarging prostate glands. This may be combined with pygeum, lysine, stinging nettle, zinc, pumpkin seed, l-glutamic acid, glycine and other agents that seem to also be beneficial.. Often this approach is sufficiently helpful that prostate surgery is not needed.

A 1998 review of 18 clinical trials of saw palmetto found that 75% of men who used saw palmetto for two months reported an improvement in their urinary symptoms.

This product can be obtained in most health food stores and through *Natural Health Team* 800-416-2806.

Cancer Of The Prostrate Gland

This was discussed in detail in the Chapter 14 on Malignancy. My personal choice of treatment for this would be flax oil and cottage cheese.

Chapter 31

Women's Health Issues

All women in developed industrial nations have an excessive exposure to estrogen, which leads to a condition referred to as estrogen dominance. This afflicts males as well as females. Estrogen dominance occurs when there is excess estrogen, decreased progesterone or when synthetic estrogen (Premarin) is used.

In an estrogen excess state, the woman may complain of bloating, salt retention with fluid gain, depression, decreased libido, fibroids, impaired blood sugar control, reduced cellular oxygen levels, increased clotting of blood, increase in body fat, and an increased risk of breast and uterine cancer.

Environmental compounds called xenoestrogens are common sources of estrogen that men and women in industrialized developed nations are exposed to. These substances, primarily of petrochemical origin, have potent estrogen like activity and are found in our air, fuels, herbicides, pesticides, plastics, clothing, propylene glycol and sodium laurel sulfate.

Propylene glycol is a common component of anti-freeze, which is also used as a solvent for flavors, extracts, drugs, antioxidant in food, emollient, humectant, for tobacco, and may be found in baked goods and coconut products.

Sodium laurelsulfate (SLS) is used in antiseptic gels, hairdressings, sunscreens, moisturizing cream, hair sprays, cosmetics, toothpaste, shampoo, and mouthwashes. SLS is a surfactant, which cleans skin and hair and creates bubbles. SLS is widely used in shampoo; bubble baths, skin care, coloring, cosmetics and body wash products.

Surfactants remain on the skin and hair long after they are presumed to have been washed off. *This causes fatty acids, moisture, and amino acids to disappear from the skin leading to dry, rough skin that has difficulty replacing old skin with new skin.* This sodium lauryl sulfate, when used, may react with other nitrogen containing chemicals to produce nitrosamines, which are carcinogens. Thus each shampoo can expose the user to the same amount of nitrates produced by eating a large amount of bacon when these nitrates are absorbed through the skin of the scalp.

Many surfactants actually injure hair follicles, which contributes to hair loss. They can injure the eyes as well by interfering with proper production of proteins in the eye after they have been absorbed through the skin and transported to the eyes.

When SLS is treated with ethylene oxide it becomes ethoxylated and is renamed sodium laureth sulfate. When used, sodium laureth sulfate creates a carcinogen named 1,4 dioxane. Dr. John Baily, the director of Colors and Cosmetics for the FDA, relates that bubble baths, shampoos, creams and lotions containing SLS have excessively high levels of 1,4 dioxane. Babies should not be in contact with these substances, as their skin is more permeable than adult skin to chemicals.

Female offspring of both animals and humans that have been exposed to xenoestrogens will be progesterone deficient. This occurs in all nations having many cars, trucks, and factories.

The American diet is contaminated with hormones. Synthetic estrogens are used to fatten cattle, chickens and other meat-producing animals. They are also used to increase milk and egg production.

Women are using more synthetic estrogens. Estrogen dominance is exacerbated by the use of synthetic estrogens from birth control pills or hormone replacement. *These synthetics estrogens are unnatural and have far more powerful effects in the body than do natural hormones.*

Progesterone levels fall in many estrogen dominant females 10 to 15 years before menopause. This results in anovulatory menstrual cycles. In an anovulatory cycle no ovulation occurs and thus *no progesterone is produced by the ovary*. This may result in heavy bleeding that can lead to hysterectomy.

Following menopause the fat cells, adrenal gland, and ovaries do continue to make estrogen at about 40% of the usual rate. *This makes the estrogen dominance even worse as progesterone levels experience a drastic fall to zero or only 1/120 of the normal level.*

When progesterone is present in the proper quantity, balanced with estrogen, there is protection against fibrocystic disease of the breast, fibroids do not enlarge, libido remains normal, fat is correctly burned for energy, blood sugar values stay normal clotting of blood remains normal, fluid is not retained, normal cellular oxygen levels are maintained and there is protection against both uterine and breast cancer.

Osteoporosis

Estrogen inhibits the osteoclast cell in bones, which dissolve old or imperfect bone. Progesterone controls the osteoblast cell, which is involved with the production of bone. Estrogen is able to slow the destruction of old or impaired bone *whereas progesterone helps build new bone*. With estrogen you are preserving the remaining fragments of bone. *With natural progesterone you are creating new bone.*

Natural progesterone produces a 10% increase in bone density within 6 months in persons with osteoporosis along with disappearance of new bone fractures. *With natural progesterone osteoporosis appears to be reversible.*

Pre-Menstrual Syndrome (PMS)

The world expert on this condition is the English physician, Dr. Katharina Dalton. She noted that her migraine headaches, which appeared with each menstruation, were gone during the last 6 months of her pregnancy. Believing that high levels of progesterone during the later stages of pregnancy had eliminated the migraine headaches, she started injecting herself with daily progesterone. The migraine headaches immediately ceased.

In a normal menstrual cycle estrogen and progesterone rise immediately after ovulation and continue to increase until menstruation begins. During this period progesterone acts as an antagonist for estrogen and negates the adverse effects of estrogen. Progesterone prepares the uterine lining to receive an impregnated ovum. If pregnancy develops the production of progesterone continues but is largely provided by the placenta instead of the ovary. If there is no pregnancy, the sudden drop in progesterone leads to shedding of the lining cells of the uterus (menstruation).

Natural progesterone is made from disgenin, a substance derived from wild yams and soybeans. *When applied to the skin this is an exact replica of the progesterone made in the body.* This is best used as a cream, which is absorbed directly into the bloodstream.

The extract of wild yams is often strong enough to correct mild hormone imbalances. When a *severe* hormone imbalance is present this will not be adequate and disgenin must be added to increase progesterone activity. *Natural progesterone is unusually safe with no known side effects discovered even after many years of usage.*

Synthetic progesterone (progestins or PROVERA) cause fluid retention, blood clots, uterine and breast cancers and emotional upsets. The problem is not really caused by hormone replacement, but *by the use of synthetic hormones.* The natural progesterone, in contrast, causes a calming effect and prevents depression.

If there is an inadequate amount of progesterone produced the following problems appear:

- Salt and Water Retention

- Low blood sugar

- Blood clotting

- Growth and Appearance of Uterine Fibroids

- Interference with thyroid function

- Increased Blood and Body Fat

- Allergic Reactions

- Loss of Zinc

- Reduced Oxygen Levels in Cells

- Endometriosis

- Fibrocystic Changes in Breast Tissue

In the most common type of premenstrual syndrome progesterone levels are low. This is associated with too much estrogen. Five reasons for estrogen excess are known:

Overproduction of Estrogen

Ovarian cysts or tumors can lead to increased estrogen production as can stress but *the most common cause is obesity. In the obese female androgen hormones are converted to estrogen.* This can only be corrected by weight loss.

The body fails to break down or remove excess estrogen.

The liver usually deactivates excess estrogen and this is secreted into the gut. Failure of this deactivation to properly occur can be brought about by liver disease or malfunction of the large bowel. Cirrhosis can increase estrogen levels.

Deficiency of nutrients can also cause problems. Pyridoxine B 6 and magnesium are necessary for the liver to neutralize estrogen. This has led to pyridoxine becoming the first therapy used in PMS. Therapy with 100 mg. of pyridoxine and 400 to 800 mg. of magnesium is recommended. The magnesium deficiency seen in PMS is caused by excessive consumption of dairy products.

Magnesium absorption is hindered by a high intake of dairy products.

These women with PMS have been found to consume three times as much refined sugar as persons with the other types of PMS. Sugar increases the excretion of magnesium and interferes with the liver's ability to deactivate estrogen. Changing the diet to one with more protein and no refined sugar increases the clearance of estrogen and prolongs the effect of progesterone.

After inactivation by the liver, estrogen goes to the intestinal tract. High fiber foods bind to this estrogen and facilitate its elimination from the body.

PMS victims need to increase the fiber in their diet and reduce their intake of animal fat. *Animal fat stimulates the growth of bacteria that can act on estrogen and permit it to be reabsorbed into the body. Furthermore, animal fats help form Prostaglandin F 2 –alpha, which decreases progesterone production by the ovary.*

This increased ability to deactivate and eliminate excess estrogen explains why women on high fiber vegetarian diets have much less PMS and less breast cancer than women on low fiber, high animal fat diets.

Bromelain may relieve menstrual cramping and also decreases the synthesis of prostaglandin F 2 alpha and increases the secretion of beneficial E 1 prostaglandin.

Excessive Breakdown of Progesterone

Physical and emotional stress promotes breakdown or conversion of progesterone into other substances.

Estrogen Supplementation Without the Addition of Natural Progesterone.

This is a frequent occurrence. Many physicians prescribe estrogen with no progesterone or synthetic progesterone, which causes problems. *Synthetic estrogen inhibits the blood concentration of natural progesterone and thus increases the female dominance with a corresponding worsening of the patients' symptoms.*

Inadequate Production of Progesterone.

The non-pregnant female produces progesterone from the corpus luteum of the ovary. PMS patients generally are lacking the nutrients that would permit an adequate amount of progesterone to be produced.

Taking 150 IU of Vitamin E increases progesterone levels.

Premenstrual Syndrome is relieved in more than 90% of patients by natural progesterone. *Synthetic estrogen may make the symptoms of PMS worse.* The synthetic estrogen inhibits the concentration of natural progesterone in the blood, which makes PMS worse by increasing estrogen dominance.

When both estrogen and progesterone are low, estrogen dominates. As previously explained, that is not good. This makes it vital to keep progesterone levels up with natural progesterone. *Uterine fibroids will not enlarge or develop and fewer hysterectomies will be needed when natural progesterone is replaced instead of estrogen.*

Researcher Dr. Raymond F. Peat relates that progesterone protects against the blood-clotting tendency caused by estrogen excess. Progesterone also appears to protect against coronary artery spasm, which helps explain why women have fewer heart attacks than men as long as their ovaries are still functioning. Progesterone also seems to play a role in regenerating damaged brain cells and prolonged growth of the brain. Delayed aging and longer life span are clearly related to extra progesterone. Many different tumors are prevented and helped by progesterone.

Progesterone and thyroid hormone regulate metabolism and appear to normalize the function of the pituitary gland. By improving oxygenation progesterone protects against low blood sugar.

Impressive studies have suggested that supplemental natural progesterone during pregnancy has the potential to produce children with higher IQ, (35 point rise) and better-adjusted personalities.

If you desire more information about this, please contact Mr. A. Tosti, Editor of Bio/Tech News, P.O.Box 30568 Parkrose Center, Portland, Oregon 97230.

Taking a natural progesterone (Dr.'s Pride Pure-Gest) can be very beneficial for PMS, menopause, and osteoporosis. This substance is obtained from the Mexican yam and contains aloe vera, Vitamin E and a vegetable base. Topical application rapidly raises progesterone levels. Application sites need to be rotated.

For most women with premenstrual syndrome, apply the progesterone cream twice daily for two months.

(In the morning when getting out of bed and at bedtime). The week before menstruation, the cream may be applied 5 times daily to curtail premenstrual symptoms. Stop the cream when menstruation begins. Use 1/4 to 1/2 teaspoon applied to the back of the neck, chest, abdomen or face. Improvement should be seen by the third month. When improvement is present, apply the cream for only one week before the suspected onset of menstruation. Take more cream if there are still symptoms or severe cramping. Many women are able to discontinue the cream after 3 or 4 months, while others continue to use it a few days each month.

Menopause

Pharmaceutical companies are unable to develop, own and sell natural products because they cannot be patented. Because of this these companies will chemically modify the natural product so they are able to obtain a patent. This produces problems *because the chemically modified compound is never as valuable as the original natural substance and usually has unwanted side effects.*

In this manner, human identical progesterone will have its molecular structure altered to create a product that *can* be patented (progestin *Provera*). This new commercial product *reverses* many of the benefits of the natural progesterone because it decreases HDL (good cholesterol), increases insulin resistance (changes carbohydrate metabolism toward becoming a diabetic), and inhibits the responsiveness of arteries by 50% (undesirable).

An Italian research study treated postmenopausal women for four weeks with estrogen then added natural progesterone to the estrogen. Exercise stress testing was performed before and after adding natural progesterone. Using estrogen alone, the women exhibited an increased capability to exert, compared to before estrogen was started. After natural progesterone was added, the women showed further improvement in their exercise capability.

When the women were given progestin (synthetic progesterone *Provera*), there was a dramatic fall in their exercise performance.

Women in their 30's under the influence of excessive estrogen tend to have anovulatory menstrual cycles. Because there is no ovulation, the ovaries produce no progesterone. During these menstrual cycles, the estrogen dominance often leads to prolonged heavy menstrual bleeding. *Most women are progesterone deficient for 10 or 15 years prior to menopause.*

For many years, I routinely prescribed Premarin and Provera. As with thousands of other doctors, I was "programmed" towards the pharmaceutical companies. To me, they had every answer. Today's indoctrination of the medical profession in favor of pharmaceutical drugs *to the total exclusion of everything else* is thorough.

Natural progesterone has several actions that protect against breast cancer. Artificial progesterone causes a marked increase in the risk of breast cancer when it is used. Despite this information, synthetic progesterone (*Provera*) is widely used by physicians.

There are three natural estrogens produced in the female (estrone, estradiol, and estriol). The widely used estrogen replacement is Premarin (conjugated estrogen), a combination of estrone, an estrogen that has been implicated in hormone related cancers, and horse hormones. Estradiol is secreted from the ovary and is a strong estrogen. Both estradiol and estrone are known to stimulate proliferation (rapid growth of breast cells), which can possibly lead to breast cancer.

Estriol is the weakest of the three natural estrogens. This has been widely used in Europe to treat menopause. Estriol has two desirable properties:

Estriol does not cause proliferation of the endometrium and thus does not cause menstrual bleeding.

Estriol has not caused the appearance of breast cancer. The doses used are 2 to 8 mg. daily, with better responses generally seen in those getting higher doses.

Another substance helps women with hot flashes. This is the herb Black Cohash, which works as well as estrogen *and has fewer side effects.* 1.7 million women routinely use this in Europe where it has the name *Remifemin.*

Natural progesterone decreases the production of a cancer causing estrogen named 4-hydroxy-estrone, while at the same time it raises the output of cancer preventing estriol.

Important research has shown that if a woman has breast cancer surgery during the luteal phase of her cycle (after ovulation and before menstruation) the survival rate is improved.

For women at onset of menopause, natural progesterone can often eliminate hot flashes. The usual medical approach is to add estrogen (Premarin) knowing that estrogen production by the ovary is falling. *This creates a problem, as the woman is already in a state of estrogen dominance and the abnormal synthetic estrogen (Premarin) increases the risk for fibrocystic breasts, fluid retention, uterine fibroid increase in size or starting to develop, uterine cancer, and an increased risk of breast cancer. (A 30% greater risk after 5 years of usage, according to Dr. John R. Lee) .*

Increasing the progesterone levels which are relatively declining far more than estrogen *with natural progesterone* will be more effective than use of estrogen and helps to reverse the problem of estrogen dominance.

Women in developed nations are estrogen dominant. Because estrogen post-menopausal is still produced in the adrenal glands, fat and ovaries at

40% of the usual amounts while progesterone output is going to zero, *women do not need estrogen replacement at menopause. The use of estrogen may even make symptoms worse.*

Occasionally a woman will develop shrinkage of the vagina associated with loss of support for the vagina and bladder. In this state of profound homone deficiency the lining membranes in the vagina are very thin. This makes intercourse impossible or painful. These women will benefit from the natural estrogen estriol which does not cause vaginal bleeding or uterine and breast cancer. The estriol should be taken along with natural progesterone.

Apply ½ to ¾ teaspoon of Dr.'s Pride Pure-Gest four times in the hour after a hot flash, which will usually stop this problem. To totally eliminate hot flashes may take from one week to several months.

Dr.'s Pride Pure-Gest is available from Bio Nutritional Formulas Inc. (800) 950 8484 and from *Natural Health Team.*

Vaginal Infections (Vaginitis)

Vaginal infections are a common problem for women. There are three categories (yeast or candida, trichomonas and bacterial).

Yeast infections often appear in women after a course of antibiotics. In the healthy situation the yeast organism are causing no problems because the healthy vaginal bacteria are dominant and able to keep the yeast from increasing. When antibiotics are given this balance is disturbed by the killing of the healthy vaginal bacteria from the antibiotic.

This leads to the multiplication of yeast in the vagina and a vaginal discharge resembling curds of milk appears along with itching in the vagina and adjacent skin. Yeast vaginal infections also frequently occur in diabetics and those on oral contraceptive therapy.

Trichomonas infection usually has a profuse frothy discharge often associated with annoying itching. This condition can be spread sexually and the sexual partner should be treated at the same time.

Bacterial vaginitis is usually the proper diagnosis if neither yeast or trichomonas are seen in the vaginal secretions. This discharge may have a peculiar fishy odor. The disease is associated with growth of gardnerella bacteria in 90% of the cases when cultures are obtained. Each of these conditions requires a different specific therapy.

Dr. Marcial-Vega has had considerable favorable experience treating all forms of vaginitis with a herbal preparation called Fem-Clenz. All the herbal preparations recommended by Dr. Vega are formulated in a water base, as the genetic DNA of herbs is injured by alcohol tincture, tablets and capsules, *none of which preserve the herbal DNA as well as water.*

One ounce of Fem-Clenz is diluted with two ounces of water and placed in the vagina daily at bedtime for one week. Dr. Marcial-Vega relates that *this is 100% effective in eliminating all forms of vaginitis.*

Fem-Clenz is available from Health Horizons 305 442-1233 or 1 800 771 -0255 and from our *Natural Health Team* 800-416-2806..

Chapter 32

Diseases Of The Nervous System

Brain Injury And Spinal Cord Injury

Physicians around the world have found DMSO to be invaluable in treating head injuries and injury to the spinal cord. Use of DMSO within a few hours of brain injuries and within one hour of injury to the spinal cord, has prevented death and paralysis that often ensues. *No other therapy is better at reducing increased intra-cranial pressure.* When head or spinal cord trauma occurs because there is bone surrounding these two structures, the fluid from the inflammatory reaction greatly increases damage to the brain and cord.

A recent study in Turkey was very interesting. Ten patients with bad head injuries were given DMSO intravenously. Their elevated intra-cranial pressure fell within 6 hours and was normal by the 6th day. Two died of their injuries, but only one of the remaining 8 had a serious neurologic deficit, when evaluated at 3 months. This is a superb result. Liberal frequent application of DMSO to the skin would probably work for a person in the USA where intravenous DMSO may not be readily available.

DMSO can be purchased from Omaha Vaccine 800 367 4444. This is a product that could be valuable in your medicine cabinet, as you cannot get it immediately in case of a stroke, head injury or spinal cord injury.

Tinnitus (Ringing In The Ears)

Tinnitus is a very annoying problem for the unfortunate persons suffering from this condition, as there is no good drug treatment for this problem.

A study published in the Annals of the New York Academy of Sciences 75; 243:468 to 474, evaluated DMSO in treating tinnitus. Patients were given 2 ml. of DMSO combined with an anti-inflammatory and a vaso-dilating agent into the auditory canals every 4 days, along with an intramuscular injection of DMSO. After one month, the tinnitus disappeared in 9 patients and was diminished in two patients and in the other two it was intermittent, instead of continuous. This is the only effective therapy for tinnitus that I am aware of.

Peripheral Neuritis

A vexing problem seen frequently by neurologists is peripheral neuritis. This condition is often manifested in the patient by pain in the extremities, weakness and loss of sensation. Frequently, neuritic pain is worse at night, preventing sleep.

The most common form of peripheral neuritis is diabetic polyneuritis, with alcoholic neuropathy also a frequent problem.

Because high dosages of alpha lipoic acid are able to reverse some cases of diabetic neuropathy, I believe that it would be reasonable to try this treatment in cases of alcoholic neuritis, as well as any case of neuritis of unknown cause, which unfortunately afflicts many more people. The dose needs to be 600 mg daily or more. (See Chapter 5).

Borage Oil

Dr. Julian Whitaker had a patient with a peripheral neuritis of unknown cause. This patient began to take gamma linolenic acid in the form of borage oil. His neuritis promptly improved with complete recovery. If it helps one person with peripheral neuritis, it might well help others. Consider giving it a try. You might even try this along with alpha lipoic acid, which also can help a peripheral neuritis. *As with many natural substances, there are no known side effects.*

Migraine Headaches

Migraine headaches are a common problem and lead to much disability, resulting in loss of work and inability to function due to severe frequent headaches.

Glucosamine Therapy

A patient with arthritis was treated with glucosamine, 500 mg twice daily. When her arthritis failed to respond her physician suggested stopping the glucosamine. *She refused because, while taking glucosamine 500 mg twice daily, her migraine headaches had ceased. This was the first headache relief from migraine that she had experienced in 20 years.*

Another physician in Australia had noted a similar experience in one of his patients on 500 mg. of glucosamine three times daily.

What percentage of migraine sufferers will benefit is not clear. A study was done by Dr. Allan Russell of Canada in 10 of his patients with difficult types of migraine. These patients were given 500 mg of glucosamine three times daily. After a lag period of 4 to 6 weeks, a worthwhile diminution in frequency and or intensity of headaches was noted. In some patients, the benefit did not appear until the dose was increased above 1500 mg daily.

If you have migraine and are not doing well, two or three months of glucosamine might be worth a try. Again, like most *natural* substances, there are no known side effects. This is available in health food stores.

Should Dental Amalgams (Mercury) Be Removed?

Dental amalgams are 50% mercury. There is a huge controversy within the dental profession about whether dental fillings are dangerous. Mercury is known to produce birth defects in newborns when the mother is exposed to mercury during pregnancy. Currently there are 1500 dentists in the U.S. who advocate removal of silver amalgams and replacement with another material.

Symptoms that can appear after exposure to mercury include seizures, muscle tremors, chronic fatigue, memory loss, depression, food and chemical sensitivities, stomach, bowel, and bladder symptoms, headache, and numbness or tingling.

In a 1998 study from the Karolinska Institute amalgam removal was followed in 60 days by a 60% fall in mercury levels in blood, plasma, and urine. With the passage of time the levels returned to those of persons who never had silver amalgams.

Evaluation of 60 patients in Sweden who had amalgam removal revealed that 78% were satisfied or very satisfied and 9.5% were disappointed. The reasons for removal varied from desire to avoid future health problems to treatment of serious current disease.

The most distressing symptoms were headache, backache, fatigue, and memory and concentration problems. Headache and backache responded best to this treatment but on average all symptoms showed considerable improvement.

At the Huggins Diagnostic Center, 85% of patients having their amalgams removed responded positively. Among the effects observed were decreased white blood cell counts in three persons that returned to normal after amalgam removal. The white cell count again became depressed when the silver amalgams were replaced. White cells are instrumental in fighting viruses, bacteria, and parasites.

Dr. Huggins tells of an 11 year old girl who was having seizures every 15 minutes, which prevented her from standing, walking or talking. Following removal of three fillings her seizures stopped in 5 days and have not returned.

A 48 year old woman with 38 amalgams had lupus erythematosus, visual problems, gastrointestinal problems, and skin rashes. These fillings were removed over a three-month period and *5 months later all her symptoms were gone.*

A commercial airline pilot developed problems with his vision and walking which led to a diagnosis of multiple sclerosis (MS). His pilot's license was in jeopardy. Following removal of 15 amalgams he experienced rapid improvement in vision, balance, and ability to walk. Many individuals have noted the disappearance of multiple sclerosis symptoms after removal of mercury amalgams.

The factors which lead to leaching of mercury from fillings include the physical stress of chewing, acidity and temperature of food and beverages, electrical currents set up between other metals in the mouth, and the act of brushing. Each surface of an amalgam leaches 1 microgram of mercury daily. Many studies have shown that the mercury content of 5 and 10 year old fillings is reduced to 25 to 30% of the original.

A study from Denmark revealed that dental clinics with seperators released 35 mg. of mercury daily whereas clinics not having seperators released 270 mg. of mercury daily. The conclusion was that dental clinics release significant amounts of mercury daily which contaminates waste water. Most U.S. clinics do not have seperators. Considering that there are 100,000 dental offices in the U.S. this would account for 12,000 pounds of mercury entering waste water annually.

However, the total mercury discharge from homes is greater than dental offices as the average person with amalgams excretes 100 micrograms of mercury daily. For the U.S. this amounts to more than 8 tons of mercury each year.

Persons with amalgams release 15.6 times more mercury into the expired air after chewing than do individuals without amalgams. Persons who chew gum release twice as much mercury from their amalgams as those who do not chew gum.

During the lifetime of an amalgam mercury vapor, ions, and particles are being inhaled and swallowed as well as being directly absorbed by the oral and nasal surfaces. Dental amalgam has been shown in human experiments to be the major source for mercury contamination of humans.

When an amalgam releases mercury the inhaled fumes can go throughout the body and reach the brain. From the nasal membranes the mercury can go directly to the pituitary gland and brain.

A research study was done in pregnant sheep. Mercury amalgams with radioactive tags were placed in molars in mid pregnancy. By the third day mercury was found in maternal and fetal blood, amniotic fluid, and maternal urine and feces.

Maternal mercury levels were highest in the kidneys, liver, g.i. tract, and thyroid gland at 16 days. At the same time sheep fetal levels were highest in pituitary gland, liver, kidneys, and placenta. By the 33rd day the mercury levels in the fetal tissues were higher than in the mother. At 73 days the mercury levels in the mother's tissues had continued to rise. These researchers felt this study showed that dental amalgam was probably the major source for human mercury exposure.

When mothers realize that their fillings can injure their baby's brains and that low I.Q. and slow learning may be a consequence they will be very upset. Mercury vapor is toxic to the fetal brain resulting in autism, attention deficit disorder, and learning disabilities.

Mercury vapor is attracted to the pituitary gland which is only one inch away from the oral cavity. It can pass directly along nerve sheaths to the brain. This concentration of mercury in the pituitary gland leads to decreased transport of oxygen and essential nutrients including amino acids, glucose, magnesium, zinc, and vitamin B 12. Depression of the enzyme isocitric dehydrogenase causes reduced iron uptake and underactive thyroid gland function, learning disability, and reduced I.Q.

The problem with mercury during pregnancy is worsened by either placing amalgams or removing amalgams during the first trimester.

Mercury is responsible for reproductive disorders including sterility, reduced fertility, and spontaneous abortions. The pituitary dysfunction from mercury can cause hormonal problems and abnormal menstrual cycles which correct after amalgam removal with improved fertility.

A study be Dr. David Eggleston of California and Dr. Magnus Nylander of Sweden in 1987 showed a direct correlation between the number of molars with amalgams and the quantity of mercury in the brain in specimens obtained from 83 cadavers. Subjects with five or more amalgams had three times more mercury than those with no amalgams.

An autopsy study of brains from patients with Alzheimer's Disease(A.D.) ten years ago disclosed that A.D. patients had double the concentration of mercury compared to patients dying of other causes. Rats exposed to levels of mercury similar to that found in the mouth of persons with high numbers of amalgams caused rapid death of the animals. The brain lesions seen were identical to those in Alzheimer's Disease.

There can be no doubt that mercury from amalgams has the potential to injure brain tissue. There is also strong evidence that aluminum is very likely incriminated in the causation of Alzheimer's Disease. This was discussed in greater detail in Chapter 26 Dementia.

At this point an important biologic concept needs to be discussed. A study from the Journal of Occuptional Toxicology revealed that laboratory rats when exposed to LDL(lethal dose level of a substance that would kill one percent of the animal population) of both lead and mercury would result in a kill rate of not two percent but nearly all the rats failed to survive.

This suggests that there is an exponential increment in the lethal effects of these metallic poisons when both were applied simultaneously. In this way the person who is leaching mercury from his dental fillings at the same time he is eating, drinking, and breathing aluminum has a greatly magnified chance of developing A.D. Whether this occurs in humans is not known to me but it might.

Additionally mercury has a harmful effect on the immune system. Mercury decreases the number of T cells. These cells diminish when amalgams are placed in the mouth and are restored when the amalgams are removed. This damage to the immune system could be responsible for permitting a minor disease or illness to become fatal.

Among the mental symptoms that can be seen with mercury exposure are irritability, anxiety, profound fatigue, depression, difficulty making trivial decisions, and impaired memory. One year after having amalgams removed 70% of these symptoms had either receded or disappeared in a study by Dr. Silberud at Colorado State University in 1988.

Are there any ill effects on dentists and dental personnel from exposure to mercury?

In 1995 behavioral testing disclosed significant impairment of concentration, emotional lability, somatosensory irritation, and mood in dentists working with mercury when compared to non amalgam exposed dentists. The urinary concentration of mercury was seven times greater in amalgam working dentists than the level found in non amalgam dentists.

Long term exposure to amalgam can cause shakiness of hands and impaired manual dexterity.

Women who worked preparing 30 or more amalgams weekly were 50 per cent less likely to conceive than unexposed women.

To me the evidence is clear that silver amalgams should no longer be placed and that persons with these amalgams should strongly consider having them replaced with ceramic amalgams. Some persons for financial or impaired health reasons may wish to postpone or not have amalgam removal. Removal of mercury prior to proceeding with amalgam removal is a good idea which makes massive release of mercury from amalgam removal less likely.

Dr. Victor Marcial-Vega of Health Horizons Clinic in Coral Gables, Florida is on the cutting edge in the development of new products to improve health care. Dr. Marcial-Vega is a board certified specialist in Radiation Oncology. His background in physics has enabled him to evaluate and create new products in a unique manner. He has co-developed a product for use in oral removal of toxic substances (NDF Non-colloidal Detox Factors) that has great merit.

This product is not a drug and should be considered a dietary supplement. The product has a special system to deliver organic whole foods in a manner that binds metals, toxins, and supports the immune system. There is synergy between the noncolloidal state of the ingredients and the delivery system permits ultra penetration of the supplement and greatly increases the bioavailability of the product. *The main use of this product is to remove toxic heavy metals from the body.*

Because the active ingredients are available in a nanocolloidal form there is a one million fold increase in the available surface area of the product. This dramatic decrease in particle size makes each ingredient more bioavailable and more effective. This means that the effective bioavailable dose is one millionth of the dose needed from the original ingredient. These particles are only .1 micron in size which enables them to easily pass through the blood brain barrier. *This permits the particles to reach tissue and intracellular areas that could not have been reached by the original ingredient.* This supplement can be absorbed via skin, oral mucosa, and intestines. Most persons with toxins have impaired assimilation and utilization of ingredients and *are unable to benefit from large molecules.*

This supplement provides nutrients for detoxification and elimination, immune support enzymes and ionic trace minerals for utilization.

Only three whole food, organic, ingredients have been selected based on in vitro heavy metal testing of metal binding capacity, positive results obtained from other supplements, and new available research on probiotics and their ferments.

Ingredients

-Nanocolloidal cell wall Chlorella Pyrenoidosa

-Nanocolloidal cilantro

-Nanocolloidal PolyFlor which contains complex ferments, cell wall lysates and enzymes from bebeficial bacteria including Bacteriocins, hyluronidase, naturally occurring Vitamin B complex, super oxide desmutase, lipoic acid, cell wall lipopoly saccharide-glycopeptide complexes, and whole peptidyl glycans.

-Pure Water containing 75 mg/liter of nanocolloidal silica

-Grain neutral spirits 20% as a preservative

-Living Water delivery system.

-BioPhoton Excitation Process

PolyFlor, Living Water, and BioPhoton Excitation Process are patented.

Poly-Flor microorganisms include 12 strains of lactobacilli(including casei, acidophilus, salivarius, bulgaris, sporogones, and plantarum), 3 strains of bifidobacterium including longum, and bifidum, and streptococcus thermophilus. b. subtilis, b. laterosporus, saccaromyces boulardil, and saccaromyces cerveciae.

Why Nanonize The Ingredients?

Chlorella has been known from mining to bind heavy metals to its cell wall. The problem with chlorella is that it has been very hard to break the cell wall. After nanonization and centrifugation there are millions of scintillating particles of .1micron size chlorella surrounded by a haze of even smaller particles.

This form of Chlorella binds to heavy metals and increases the elimination of toxins, regulates growth hormone, is a powerful nutrient and protects from radiation.

Cilantro stimulates the excretion of methyl mercury through the breath.

Poly-Flor contains complex ferments, cell wall lysates, and enzymes from beneficial bacteria. There is strong clinical evidence that beneficial lactic acid forming bacilli gut flora are effective against harmful gut flora by competitive exclusion. They also help travelers diarrhea(parasites), antibiotic induced diarrhea, radiation damage, chemotherapy, h. pylori infection, formation of carcinogens, and restore normal bowel flora.

They also stimulate the immune system in a powerful manner.

Heavy metal toxicity especially from dental amalgams leads to impaired intestinal function and candida. The complex ferments, bacteriocins, cell wall lysates, and enzymes from beneficial bacteria in NDF may prepare the intestinal terrain for restoration of normal gut flora via the mechanism of competitive exclusion. *Normal gut bacterial flora can not be established until the metals are gone.* Bacteria exposed to mercury from dental fillings are more vulnerable to developing resistance to antibiotics.

The ferments and metabolites of Poly-Flor assist the penetration of other active ingredients, bind with greater affinity to cell receptor sites than toxins, dissolve solvents, and paraffin(plaque), may restore neurologic function and a sense of well being.

A person with normal bowel flora is always better protected against environmental toxins than a person with bowel dysfunction. When amalgams are in teeth, or the toxic burden becomes too great, or when a person consumes processed foods and pesticide grown food, the powerful benefits of these agents may be overwhelmed.

The Living Water is very important. It is unused water. There are ten steps needed to make this water.

Our cells communicate with biophotons(cellular molecules and electricity) at a specific frequency of light. Toxic cells lose their biophotons to healthy cells. The BioRay proprietary preparation restores biophotons to the endangered cells. Laboratory studies have confirmed that NDF binds to heavy metals and excretes them in the urine.

Clinical Results

1.   Persons so toxic from metals that they require regular continuing intravenous chelation have remained stable and continue to improve with NDF. Laboratory studies have shown that mercuy is more effectively removed by NDF than by intravenous chelation.

2.   A 49 year- old female with a diagnosis of acute intermittent porphyria had suffered from constant abdominal pain and exhaustion for 15 years. After two weeks of therapy great improvement occurred.

Dental amalgam removal should be done by a dentist who is experienced in this procedure. We recommend that NDF be taken for at least two weeks before starting dental amalgam removal. If, because of financial, poor heath or logistical reasons amalgam extraction is impossible, NDF should be continued on a permanent basis. Probably, NDF taken one month out of every 3 or 4 months would be adequate to keep the mercury burden well controlled. Intravenous chelation is not very effective in removing mecury. We recommend NDF for all persons who have amalgams.

We think because NDF eliminates aluminum, it might be beneficial in persons with Alzheimer's Disease and certainly a two to three month trial seems reasonable. Some persons eliminate metals predominately in urine, others through stools, some through the lungs, others through sweat or by any combination of the above.

The NDF is supplied in a one half- ounce bottle. This is preserved with 20% neutral spirits. The therapy is initiated by taking one drop in a glass of water the first day. The dosage is increased by one drop each day.

Two types of toxic symptoms may appear. One of these is the odor of mercury on the breath. The second is the appearance of fever and aching suspicious of influenza. When either of these symptoms appear the drops are discontinued until the symptoms cease when therapy may be resumed. Usually these toxic symptoms appear within a few days.

Improvement in symptoms is one of the best ways to be sure you are benefiting from NDF. This therapy with NDF should be continued as long as symptoms are diminishing and the elimination of metals is improving. This may last from a few months to longer than a year. At that point the therapy may be continued as a preventative measure several times each year.

NDF is much less expensive and consumes far less time than intravenous chelation. NDF is taken orally while chelation is given intravenously over a three hour period. Chelation is given once or twice weekly for 20 to 30 treatments.

Dr. Marcial Vega has noted that patients taking NDF often notice disappearance of varicose veins. Additionally, patients with schizophrenia may become well after several months of therapy. They remain well. NDF is a food supplement which can be obtained from Health Horizon Phone 305 442-1233 or 800 771-0255 or from our *Natural Health Team* 800-4162806. Prior to shipping the NDF is placed in a scalar lab where it is given an electrical charge that lasts one year.

Effective Therapy For Cerebrovascular Disease

Padma has proven effective for cerebrovascular disease as well as coronary and peripheral vascular disease. In the neurology department at the regional hospital in Zyrardow, Poland 35 patients with cerebral arteriosclerosis were treated with Padma. Their ages ranged from 32 to 72. Nine had carotid artery blockage and fourteen had suffered either temporary blood lack to the brain (TIA) or had a stroke in the preceding two years.

All persons were given 6 tablets of Padma daily for 6 weeks, then 4 tablets daily. Nearly every patient showed improvement. Twenty five noted improved memory and the disapperance of emotional instability. Five of the nine with carotid artery narrowing lost all symptoms related to this disorder. No patient with a history of TIA had a new TIA. This represents a significant therapeutic advance. The benefits of Padma would appear to be similar to those found in patients with cerebrocascular disease after hyperbaric oxygen therapy.

Padma Basic is available from Nutri Center USA 800-701-8648 and from *Natural Health Team* 800-416-2806.

Chapter 33

Tobacco Addiction

Actuarial studies have revealed that cigarette smokers shorten their lives by 6 to 8 years, compared to nonsmokers. They have a higher incidence of sudden death and more arterial disease, emphysema, and malignancies than nonsmokers.

Cigarette smokers are three times more likely than a nonsmoker to have a stroke and more than twice as likely as a nonsmoker to have a heart attack.

The problem of sudden death immediately ceases when a smoker quits (see Chapter 3 Heart Disease). Often the lung damage from emphysema improves by 10 to 20% after cigarettes are terminated. We have seen earlier in this book how artery damage can be reversed.

How Does Nicotine Addiction Work?

Nicotine binds with neuro-receptors in the brain. When the nicotine disappears from these receptors, there is an instant demand for more nicotine.

A new product, Sulfonil, binds to these receptors and thus reduces the craving. Take 2 capsules on arising then 1 every 4 to 6 hours during the day and 2 at bedtime. This needs to be continued for from 3 days to two weeks, until the craving for a cigarette is gone. The Sulfonil needs to be supplemented with a good multivitamin, 2 quarts of water daily and mild walking. The addiction craving will be gone by two weeks, but the habit of smoking may take up to three weeks to disappear.

Anxiety Control, which can be purchased from a health food store or from Pain and Stress Center 800-669 2256, may be taken. Two pills twice daily can help. This contains aminoacids GABA, glycine, and glutamine.

Sulfonil can be obtained from Sound Nutrition 800-844 6645

Plantago Major

This plant known as the broadleaf plantain has been noted to help bronchitis. This plant was found to cause a strong aversion to tobacco when inhaled or ingested.

Twenty four heavy smokers were given a tincture of plantago major through a nasal spray and were instructed to smoke. 83% of the subjects had an immediate aversion to tobacco, which lasted from 2 to 24 hours. When an individual feels the desire to smoke, they spray the CIG-No spray onto their tongue. This creates the sensation that they have "already smoked too much". The CIG-No is safe and reportedly has no side effects. This can be obtained from M.E. Cody Inc. 800-431 2582

Noni

Noni is reported to be good therapy for tobacco addiction. It has the advantage of simplicity. Take 4 ounces of Noni twice daily for three days, which seems to be long enough to break the cigarette habit with Noni.

Noni can be obtained from Brower Enterprises or from *Natural Health Team* 800-416-2806.

Chapter 34

Suggestions For Ways To Take Natural Products

In my opinion if you try a natural substance for *two months* and can see no improvement, you can stop the substance.

It is very difficult to know *which* agent is helping you, and which agent is not working when you add more than one therapy at the same time. Sometimes, the need for a favorable response is urgent and then you may choose to start with several substances.

How can you tell if an unusual problem you are experiencing is from a substance you are taking?

The best way is to stop taking the suspected substance. If the symptom goes away and then comes back when you reintroduce this substance, you can be quite confident that you are having a reaction to this substance.

Keep your physician informed about your thoughts and ideas. Your doctor may be aware that a medicine you are taking will conflict with the natural therapy.

Noni

Noni appears to be nature's universal antidote for almost all illnesses, which made it inappropriate to place in any of the preceding chapters. It works for many different health problems. This Polynesian fruit is reliably reported to be beneficial in treating (but not curing) cancer, hypertension, Type 2 diabetes, gout, digestive disorders, infections, injuries, lung diseases, high cholesterol values, and drug and alcohol abuse.

Japanese researchers determined that an anthraquinone compound called damnacanthal found in Noni was the most active extract of 500 extracts tested against the K-ras-NRK cell, a precursor to several cancers. Noni appeared to act directly on host macrophages and lymphocytes to counteract cancer cells.

French researchers confirmed that Noni is non-toxic and that it exhibited consistent central (brain) pain relieving activity.

Most of the important research on this fascinating substance was done by Dr. Ralph Heineke. Dr. Heineke received his Ph. D. in biochemistry from the University of Minnesota. Dr. Heineke believes that much of the therapeutic benefits of Noni are related to an alkaloid called proxeronine in Noni, that becomes converted to the alkaloid xeronine in the body. He feels that the healing properties of Noni are due to this alkaloid precursor, which appears to effect cancer, lower blood pressure, heal infections, relieve arthritis, lower blood sugar, and relieve pain.

Twenty- five years ago, Dr. Heineke isolated the enzyme xeronine from bromelain. He discovered that xeronine is manufactured in small quantities in the human body and plays a critical role in the function of enzymes and proteins in the body. *Xeronine is depleted under any kind of stress.* The proneronine from Noni was readily converted to xeronine by intestinal cells full of serotonin.

Lack of xeronine disrupts the body's resistance to illness, infection, and chronic degenerative diseases. The quantity of xeronine produced declines with aging and all forms of stress (viral illness, injury, surgery, difficult occupation, worry, and anger). This may explain why high stress persons are vulnerable to more illnesses and chronic degenerative illnesses.

The happy -go -lucky individual maintains optimum xeronine levels and manages to avoid serious illnesses. When a psychologist improves an individual's mental and emotional state, any disease present may begin to improve because xeronine is no longer being stolen by the stressing incidents in the person's life. *Noni can help avoid depletion of xeronine that would ordinarily ensue from a stressful life.*

Without proper xeronine levels, vitamins do not work and serious illness may result, including cancer, premature aging, viral illness, and immune system malfunction. When a protein or enzyme fails to function properly due to low xeronine levels, every cell, tissue, and organ needing that protein or enzyme may fail (heart disease, kidney disease, diabetes). *Restoring correct xeronine levels may alleviate those diseases.*

Dr. Heineke states that xeronine is by far the best treatment for reversing hard -core drug addiction. He states, "By flooding the brain with xeronine, the proteins in the brain are changed. Within a matter of days, brand new receptor sites are created due to xeronine's work on proteins. *Now you have normal receptor sites in the brain that respond to xeronine instead of drugs*".

Nicotine addiction can be cured in three days by the same mechanism.

Noni And Pain

Many people use DMSO to relieve pain. DMSO is unable to relieve pain adequately because it is a simple solvent. When DMSO is applied to the skin, it releases the skin xeronine, which gets transported deeper to the painful area where it affects cells, relieving the pain.

DMSO often acts wonderfully the first time it is applied, but works less well the second time and perhaps not at all on third application, because all the skin xeronine is gone. Time will be needed for restoring skin xeronine.

Case Reports

A breast cancer patient in France refused surgery and was placed on xeronine three times daily. The patient made a complete recovery.

A male patient became impotent and developed a rash while taking cholesterol-lowering medicine. When switched to xeronine, his cholesterol values became normal and his potency returned.

A woman in Tahiti with cancer was given only to weeks to live. A Tahitian friend urged her to try Noni, which she did resulting in complete recovery. There is no guaranteed cure for cancer. However it has helped some individuals.

A colleague of Dr. Heineke gave proxeronine (NONI's active alkaloid) to a woman who had been comatose for three months. *Two hours later she sat up and asked where she was.*

My personal knowledge of Noni is fascinating. An elderly man developed trouble walking and became confined to bed. His physician advised him that there was no medical treatment for this problem and that he would die soon. He started taking Noni, regained his ability to walk and was in good health one year later.

A 55 year- old male with insulin requiring diabetes gained 35 pounds after going on insulin therapy. He started Noni and lost 25 pounds over a 6 week period. Additionally, his blood sugars have shown significant improvement.

For one month I had been troubled by a deep right lower abdominal aching that occurred several time daily, lasting about one minute. This pain seemed to me like it might be from seminal vesiculitis, because it radiated into the right side of the scrotum. This pain immediately ceased after starting Noni. Because Noni benefits both pain and infections, it was impossible to be certain which was being corrected.

Taking Noni regularly keeps body xeronine levels intact and strengthens defenses against chronic degenerative disease. As with most natural products, there are no known side effects. I think Noni might be beneficial in patients with drug-resistant tuberculosis, osteomyelitis and HIV.

The dose of Noni is one or two ounces daily, but may need to be increased to three or four ounces daily for serious conditions.

Noni can be obtained from Brower Enterprises 800- 373 6067 and from our *Natural Health Team* 800-416-2806.

Hydrogen Peroxide Therapy

The use of intravenous hydrogen peroxide therapy nearly ceased with the advent of antibiotics, which is unfortunate. In 1920 Doctors Oliver and Cantab reported in Lancet about their experiences in treating pneumonia with intravenous hydrogen peroxide. They were fighting a pneumonia outbreak in Indian troops that was killing 80% of it's victims. They gave intravenous hydrogen peroxide to cases they felt were hopeless. Of these hopeless cases 13 out of 25 survived.

Two Indian doctors created gas gangrene infections in dogs. Both groups of dogs were given 2 billion gas forming bacteria into the muscles of their legs.

One group received hydrogen peroxide into the artery going to the leg and the other received no therapy. The untreated animals all died but 10 of the 12 animals getting hydrogen peroxide survived.

Hydrogen peroxide has recognized uses as a bleaching agent, as an antiseptic and disinfectant, as an oxidizing agent and an oxidizer for small rockets.

Injected hydrogen peroxide reacts with the enzyme catalase in plasma and white blood cells releasing oxygen. The venous blood after HP infusion takes on the same color as arterial blood because of the added oxygen content. The quantity of oxygen released is comparable to that found in a hyperbaric oxygen chamber. This is important because hyperbaric oxygen chambers are expensive to use, have some risks, and are not readily available.

Dr. Charles Farr observed that *the increased oxygen content of tissues appeared 40 to 45 minutes after the injection of HP.* This delayed rise in tissue oxygen levels suggested that the hydrogen peroxide was not immediately broken down into water and oxygen, and, thus the oxygen would not immediately be blown out of the lungs. This means the hydrogen peroxide would be distributed all over the body before releasing oxygen and *that little if any oxygen would be lost through expiration.*

The clinical benefit from the oxygen saturation of tissue fluid may be of secondary importance because very little peroxide is injected and thus *very little oxygen is produced.* Of greater importance appears to be the powerful oxidizing effects of hydrogen peroxide (HP). HP oxidizes toxic and nontoxic substances. This oxidation is valuable because *fat deposition in artery plaques can be removed.*

White blood cells are involved in killing bacteria. When white cells encounter bacteria they engulf them. The white cell creates hydrogen peroxide from oxygen and water and this HP dissolves the bacteria. This HP production is the primary defense against bacteria, viruses, parasites, and yeast. Studies have shown that hydrogen peroxide is effective in treating Legionnaire's Disease, syphilis, yeast (candida), viruses and parasites. In a hospital setting it is *imperative that oxygen therapy be stopped when hydrogen peroxide is infused because oxygen administration blocks the desired conversion of water and oxygen into hydrogen peroxide inside the cell and thus bacterial lysis does not occur.*

HP is involved in all life's vital processes including protein, carbohydrate, and fat metabolism, vitamin and mineral metabolism, and the manufacture of prostaglandins after Vitamin C administration, which benefits immunity.

Measurements of lung artery oxygen content were studied before and after HP therapy. Following infusion of HP the oxygen content rose from 60 to 80 a marked improvement.

Thirty years ago Dr. Finney and colleagues at Baylor University Medical School infused HP into leg arteries of patients with severe arteriosclerosis. This therapy clears the arteries and the improvement persisted. Autopsies performed one year later revealed that the artery clearing was still present. This appeared to be more effective than intravenous chelation, which works best on small arteries.

Hydrogen peroxide has an energizing effect on the heart (inotropic effect). This causes the heart to beat with more force and greater efficiency. One of the grave complications during a heart attack is ventricular fibrillation. The heart is beating in an ineffective manner pumping little blood.In this setting of severe oxygen lack the *emergency use of HP has reversed ventricular fibrillation certainly by providing desperately needed oxygen.*

A group of New Zealand rabbits were strangled by clamping the trachea. They all died within 12 minutes from cardiac stoppage or ventricular fibrillation. However, if the same strangled rabbits were given hydrogen peroxide into the arteries of the heart they all survived two hours without problems. This means that the arterial HP infusion was providing a perfectly satisfactory amount of oxygen to the heart. Even many of the strangled rabbits after 12 minutes could be resuscitated from imminent death by dripping HP onto the exposed heart.

Then rabbits had their arteries to the heart tied off which produces death in 5 to 10 minutes from heart stoppage or ventricular fibrillation. However, injecting HP into a peripheral vein returned their heart beating and blood pressure rapidly back to normal in most animals. *Even dripping HP directly on the heart muscle would save many of the rabbits from death.*

In the same experiments with pigs when the animals appeared dead without blood pressure or heart beating there was recovery in 50% when HP was applied to the heart.

The beneficial clearing of arterial plaque by HP was attempted in 1967 on a woman at Baylor who had blockage of the main artery(carotid) to the brain from a stroke. Surgery was performed on the right carotid artery to correct this blockage. Nine months later she subsequently developed blockage of the right vertebral artery. The vertebral arteries are in the back of the brain and are not accessible to surgery. When they become blocked dizziness, balance, vision loss and speech may be disturbed. These patients may drop to the ground without obvious reason.

A decision was made to infuse HP into the main neck arteries because blood thinning had not helped. She received 100 infusions over 28 days. In the first week her coordination and speech improved and she became able to sit up without dizziness.

Hydrogen Peroxide and Cancer

Radiation therapy does shrink tumor masses but it injures the immune system. Cancer cells cannot tolerate oxygen. The Baylor team decided to inject HP into the artery going to the tumor while simultaneously using radiation therapy.

Case 1 An 88 year old man with squamous call cancer of his right cheek received HP dripped into his right carotid artery along with radiation. Six years later he was still well. The usual life expectancy of this tumor is 12 to 18 months.

Case 2 A 29 year old man with a cancerous mass that had fixed his tongue and caused gangrene of the jaw bone received infusion of HP along with radiation and made a complete recovery.

Are There Problems With HP Therapy?

The most frequent side effect noted is inflammation(phlebitis) of the vein used for the infusion. This is less frequent when large veins are used and less likely if slow infusions are given(one and a half hours). This clears spontaneously and is helped by *cold* compresses.

At times after HP there is massive death of bacteria occurring in a short time span. This release of large amounts of foreign material into the circulation may cause migrating aching, nausea, headache, chills but no fever (Herxsheimer reaction). It usually appears in the first three treatments and the patient continues to get well. The reaction is caused by too great a release of toxins in response to the treatment (overkill). Skin eruptions are a good sign suggesting that toxins are being released. None of the side effects are frequent.

When used in an office it is easy to monitor the effect of HP treatment. A pulse oximeter can be placed on a finger to monitor oxygen level. If there is no rise in finger oxygen during the infusion the hydrogen peroxide solution has deteriorated and needs to be replaced with fresh solution.

Can HP Therapy Be Given Orally?

This is a controversial area. Some authorities recommend oral HP while others condemn it. The enzymes that break up hydrogen peroxide into oxygen and water are lacking in the stomach which creates a situation in which oral HP may cause nausea and irritation to the stomach(ulcer). This is made more dangerous if HP is taken along with food, iron or vitamin C so it must always be taken in an empty stomach. The safest form of HP is reagent grade, which contains much less lead than USP hydrogen peroxide. Do not exceed 10 drops of 3% solution three times daily if you decide to try this.

Hydrogen Peroxide And The Immune System

Dr. Charles Farr made an astute observation those persons who have received a series of intravenous HP injections become less sensitive to pollens and food. Improvement in asthma, allergic bronchitis, and chronic sinusitis were also noted.

Farr had previously noted that patients given intravenous HP had a 55% reduction in their null(baby) lymphocytes which are destined to become B-cells and T-cells. He felt this decrease in null cells was due to increased differentiation into T-cells and B-cells. Possibly these new T-cells and B-cells *have not been exposed to the previous irritating antigens.*

Study of patients with autoimmune disorders (rheumatoid arthritis, sub acute lupus erythematosis, psoriasis, multiple sclerosis) revealed that after 10 or more intravenous infusions of HP the autoimmune antibodies that help diagnose these diseases were no longer detectable. The previously mentioned decrease in sensitized T and B cells may be the cause for clinical improvement in these diseases. Because these new T and B cell lymphocytes derived from null cells have not been tagged to produce specific antibodies, the quantity of circulating antibody falls with a corresponding clinical improvement.

Hydrogen Peroxide And Gum Disease (Gingivitis)

Dr. Weston Price, a great nutritionist, traveled the world studying health issues. He noted that native tribes in the South Pacific *that had not been exposed to modern food never got cavities or gum disease.* He concluded that the cavities were not caused by rotten food. *They are caused by a rotten diet.* His observations were confirmed by the arctic explorer Vilhajmur Stefansson.

The bad foods for teeth are sugar, fluoride, synthetic vegetable fats, and other nutrition free food substitutes.

Dr. Paul Cummings of Wilmington, North Carolina taught gingival(gum) disease at the University of North Carolina. He now recommends using hydrogen peroxide and baking soda rubbed into the diseased gums after the teeth have been professionally cleaned. He states that this program is obtaining a 98% success rate *far better than he ever obtained with surgery. Cummins relates that not one clinical study has ever shown that periodontal surgery was necessary.*

Interesting Case Reports

Mr. J.H. had received 11 chelation treatments for heart disease. On his way to get his 12th treatment he developed signs of a stroke. His speech became slurred, his vision blurred, and fluid drooled from the side of his mouth. Dr. Farr found him to be confused and disoriented. His symptoms suggested the early stage of a stroke.

Dr. Farr instantly started intravenous HP. Within 15 minutes his mind cleared and his speech improved. *One hour later he had no symptoms.*

J.O. was a 67-year-old man with severe blockage of the leg arteries and extensive blockage of his heart (coronary) arteries. He has already received bypass operations on both legs and had a 4-bypass heart operation.

Gangrene, dying tissue due to oxygen lack, was present in the left leg and he was urged to have amputation of the left leg below the knee. Previous intravenous chelation treatments had not helped. There was severe pain in the left great toe.

Dr. Farr suggested a trial of intravenous HP. His first treatment was followed by decrease in toe pain, which continued to disappear completely. He eventually lost the toe but *the leg was saved and he was able to throw away his crutches.*

M.G., a 71-year-old female, developed temporal arthritis, which is a severe inflammatory reaction in arteries often involving the scalp vessels and forehead. Sudden blindness may result. This responded to cortisone therapy, which caused ulcers, inflammation of the pancreas, and colitis.

Dr. Farr recommended a trial of HP. Her pain began to decrease during the first infusion and she became well after the second infusion.

Dr. Farr also treated a man with acute shingles (herpes zoster) involving the neck, shoulder, and right arm with HP. He was better three days later and back to normal in 7 days. *Not all cases of shingles improve with HP.*

Emphysema (chronic obstructive pulmonary disease) has been treated by Dr. Farr with good response. The patients develop a cough during the infusion, which can be terminated by slowing the infusion and it reappears when the infusion is resumed. The released oxygen is believed to seep into air pockets below the mucous in the bronchial tube lining. This mucous becomes loosened which leads to sputum production followed by improvement.

P.M. developed yeast syndrome after prolonged treatment of lung infections with antibiotics. She developed chronic vaginal infection with yeast, intermittent diarrhea, fatigue, acne, arthritis, headaches, and difficulty concentrating. The usual therapies for yeast led to temporary improvement but her symptoms always recurred.

After two intravenous HP treatments her alertness and ability to concentrate were improved along with a sense of well-being. She became symptom free after 8 infusions for the first time in eight years.

A model who was a patient of Dr. William Campbell Douglass accepted an assignment in two days in Dallas. She came in with temperature of 101 degrees F. red eyes and a red nose. Dr. Douglass started a HP infusion. She was 90% better the next day and back to normal in two days able to accept her assignment.

Mrs. J.C., a 42-year-old woman had been offered a position as a college professor, but was reluctant to take the position because of severe symptoms (fatigue, weakness, lethargy, fever, *and sluggish thought processes*) that would interfere with her job performance. Her illness began three months earlier with low-grade fever, mental lethargy, fatigue, and weakness. She had deteriorated to such an extent that getting out of bed in the morning was nearly impossible. Therapy with antibiotics and rest had accomplished nothing.

She was given intravenous Vitamin C(35grams) three times which led to slight improvement in her thought processes but the decreased fatigue after the injections lasted only 24 hours. She agreed to try HP therapy. The first intravenous infusion contained 250 cc. of 5% glucose in water with two cc of 15% hydrogen peroxide. *There was immediate benefit. Her fatigue was gone in three hours and her thought processes became clear and normal.* The next two days she received the same infusion. She took the position and has remained well. Her illness sounded like chronic fatigue syndrome with possible candida syndrome superimposed.

Mr. R.D. had terminal emphysema. He came to the office in a wheel chair with oxygen flowing from a bottle. After 4 HP treatments he discarded his oxygen and wheel chair. Terminal emphysema patients are so short of breath the mere exertion of eating is too difficult and they lose weight. *Mr. R.D. regained his appetite and gained 8 pounds.*

Patient R.T.T. had angina (chest pain from poor blood supply to the heart), uncontrolled diabetes, and fatigue. An arm fracture had failed to heal for two years.

Following HP treatments his chest pain disappeared, the diabetes came under control with normal blood sugars, and his energy dramatically increased. *To everyone's amazement the arm fracture healed.*

C.S. age 26 developed systemic lupus erythematosus with convulsions (cerebritis). She also had two episodes of kidney injury from lupus with poor kidney function. After starting on oral hydrogen peroxide she became better.

The consulting university specialists questioned the diagnosis because she had improved without taking cytoxan. Cytoxan had been refused because she knew it was dangerous. She did not tell her physician or the university specialists she was taking oral HP but they would probably not have believed it could help her anyway.

Another patient had severe herpes zoster (shingles) which left him with severe chest wall pain. This pain is occasionally so severe that patients consider suicide. Weekly infusions of HP led to complete resolution of his pain in 10 weeks.

Practical Considerations

Physicians are under pressure in their offices to do something curative for the patient who comes in with fever, aching, cough and headache. The physician is in a dilemma. He has a sick patient who wants to be well. All patients know that antibiotics cure infections and this knowledge translates into a desire to receive an antibiotic prescription. The physician is aware that 75 to 80% of these illnesses are caused by viruses and will not respond to antibiotic therapy.

The availability of HP for office use supplies the physician with an effective safe therapy that can resolve the illness immediately. This therapy will cure either viral or bacterial infection without side effects. No prescriptions are needed for an antibiotic that may produce side effects and cause antibiotic resistance to develop. My hope is that this information will cause many physicians, clinics, and hospitals to make HP available to patients.

This therapy has other important considerations. During influenza epidemics massive amounts of days are lost from work. HP will get patients well and back to work quickly saving many man-hours. Additionally, the influenza virus acts by stripping off the lining membranes from the bronchial tubes. In this denuded state of the bronchi bacteria can easily invade the lung and pneumonia of an unusually virulent type (large cavities often appear in the lung x-rays after 5 or 6 days) results.

In 1960 I was stationed at the U.S. Navy Hospital in Charleston, S.C. during an influenza epidemic. Most of the deaths during an influenza epidemic are not from the virus but are due to secondary bacterial infection. We saw young healthy males go from being well to dead with pneumonia in 48 hours. The physician must select the correct antibiotic because you get no second chance.

Now with HP this whole course can be changed. To begin with the initial presentation with fever can be cured *so pneumonia never gets a chance to occur.* Secondly, using HP, would be of inestimable value for the critically ill person with early pneumonia. This therapy will start to correct both the virus and any bacteria that have started to invade the lung. *If the antibiotic choice turns out to be wrong the patient still gets well.*

I urge physicians and hospitals to get involved with starting HP programs so lives can be saved that might otherwise be lost. This is a simple technology that is readily adapted to a physician's office. This has the potential to return healing to the physician's office, where it belongs.

The International Oxidative Medicine Association was established by Dr. Charles Farr. By making a $5 donation to this foundation at P.O. Box, 809010, Oklahoma City, OK. 73189 they will supply you with an updated list of physicians who are experienced in hydrogen peroxide therapy.

All the information about hydrogen peroxide therapy in this chapter was obtained from Dr. William Campbell Douglass's remarkable book *Hydrogen Peroxide Medical Miracle.*

What To Do Every Day To Stay Healthy

Take MULTIVITAMINS daily. They must be free of iron and contain minerals. Vitamin C should be at least 300mg. daily. Also take Vitamin E 400mg to 800mg., Beta carotene 15,000 units, Vitamin D 400IU better 800 IU, B complex, Vitamin A 5,000 units and Biotin 300mcg.

Minerals that are needed include Calcium, Iodine, Magnesium, Zinc, Copper, Manganese, Chromium, Selenium 200 mcg., Molybdenum, Vanadium and Boron.

Flaxseed Or Flax Oil

Everyone will benefit from taking 4 tablespoons of ground flaxseed or 2 tablespoons of flax oil daily. This will correct the widespread deficiency of Omega 3 essential fatty acids found in diets containing artificial substances like margarine, salad oil, and shortenings. Most foods have these artificial oils added to them.

Flax has great potential to prevent degenerative diseases and keep us healthy.

It is probable that persons who are eating a nutritious diet and taking vitamins, minerals, antioxidants and flaxseed will have a greatly reduced incidence of cancer, arteriosclerosis and arthritis.

Melatonin

Consider taking melatonin daily if you have a sleep problem. This provides a powerful antioxidant, immune supporting substance that may have longevity benefits, as well.

Noni

Take an ounce of NONI daily if you are in a stressful situation or have daily stress from your occupation.

Saw Palmetto

If you are a male, consider taking saw palmetto, 500mg to 520 mg twice daily starting at age 45 to 50. This may prevent you from having to deal with a grossly enlarged prostate gland at a later date.

N-Acetyl Cysteine

The daily intake of 600 mg. of n-acytl-cysteine will raise glutathione levels by 38%, which should greatly enhance the function of the immune system.

DHEA

Taking DHEA after age 40 may improve general health as we age. Nearly everyone over the age of 40 has low levels of DHEA-s (sulfate below 200mcg/dL). The normal values of a youth are 400mcg. to 560mcg. for males and 350mcg. to 430 mcg. for females. Obtain a blood DHEA test after 3 to 6 weeks of DHEA therapy to help regulate the correct dosage.

The usual dose is 25mg. daily for females and 50mg. daily for males. This dosage needs to be altered based on regular blood tests.

The benefits of DHEA treatment include counteracting stress, better immune function, elevation of insulin growth factor (IGF) which preserves muscles and diminishes fat accumulation, may protect against the development of heart disease, prevents against excessive clotting of blood, improves survival in population studies, helps 50 to 60% of depressed persons, usually beginning in 10 days, and protects against brain aging.

To insure protection against possible prostatic enlargement and or prostate cancer, rectal exam and PSA blood test should be done *before* initiating DHEA and annually thereafter. In addition, Vitamin E 400 to 800mg., selenium 200mcg. lycopene 20 to 40 mg., and saw palmetto

500mg. daily should help protect against the development of a prostate problem.

Women may experience rising estrogen levels with DHEA therapy. Women with estrogen dependent breast cancer must get advice from their physician before starting this treatment.

Patients with liver disease should take DHEA sublingually or in a skin cream, so less DHEA passes through the liver. Obviously, liver function should be regularly monitored.

The most effective way to reverse aging is with growth hormone. This converts fat to muscle, increases stamina and improves sexual performance. Unfortunately this is expensive but less so with secretagogue therapy than the use of intra-muscular injections of growth hormone. We recommend a trial of daily use of *Young Again*. For persons who would like a less expensive approach, the use of DHEA, as previously discussed should be beneficial. Persons taking growth hormone should not take DHEA.

Last, but extremely important, *what we eat and drink has a profound effect on our health.* Start eating lots of fruit and vegetables. Get rid of the synthetic, artificial margarine, shortenings, and salad oils, and cut back your protein intake to the 50 grams range. Try to eat fish regularly. Begin to obtain some fermented food (sauerkraut, yogurt) in a small quantity daily.

Obtain some system to filter your water.

All the above will help you maintain your health.

Epilogue

The more I have studied natural healing treatments the clearer it has become to me that the Creator of the Universe has not left mankind helpless at the mercy of a torrent of diseases and afflictions.

Man is extremely resourceful and hard working. Look at the wonderful natural substances we've already discussed. *There are certainly many more natural treatments that I know nothing about.* It is nearly impossible to find a major illness for which there is not some form of effective natural treatment.

The exciting thing about these natural treatments is that they are, in general, safe and less expensive than pharmaceutical drugs. *They certainly have far fewer side effects. They're natural and in harmony with our bodies.*

Physicians who begin to encourage their patients to try natural treatments will be delighted with the results. We of *Natural Health Team* have planned ahead and would be delighted to work with any health insurance company that wishes to initiate a natural health treatment program.

As the trend toward natural healing therapies continues, what changes might occur?

There will be an excess of hospital beds as fewer patients need hospital care. As chemotherapy declines fewer cancer patients will be in hospitals, as many of these patients will recover and stay well.

Improved management of diet and antioxidants will decrease the number of patients receiving angioplasty, stents and bypass surgery in hospitals.

Many patients with autoimmune illnesses will become well and no longer be seen in hospitals (lupus, rheumatoid arthritis, multiple sclerosis, hepatitis B and C). Hepatitis C patients will get well and not require long hospitalizations for liver transplantation.

Better control of diabetes and reversal of diabetic complications will decrease the number of diabetic patients (gangrene, stroke, heart attack, leg ulcers, infections and uremia) now staying in hospitals. Many diabetics will be cured of their illness by changing their fat intake.

Disability from hip fractures and compression fractures of the spine requiring hospitalization will be much less frequent with better prevention and correction of osteoporosis.

HIV patients will be able to stabilize their T cell lymphocyte counts so they do not fall to the low levels, where continuous life threatening infections require hospitalization.

Fewer patients with asthma will relapse and require hospital stays. Hopefully, better antibiotic programs for animals and humans will decrease the serious infections now being seen in hospitals.

Persons using essential oils will be preserved from an anthrax outbreak, exactly as the grave robbers were during the Black Death (bubonic plague).

There will be a surplus of physicians. Many of these well trained and scientifically oriented individuals will go to work for companies with natural health care products where they will be an asset in screening out substances of doubtful merit, selecting simple ways to prove performance of products and providing credibility for these companies.

Others will be needed to help insurance companies and governmental agencies provide natural health treatment programs that are up to date and full of substances that work. Many physicians will be needed to evaluate how to use natural health products and *to discover the basic mechanisms of action for many of these substances.* Biochemists, physiologists, pharmacologists and other scientific personnel will be needed to clarify how these multitudes of substances work.

Some specialties will need fewer physicians (opthalmology, oncology, allergy). *There will be steady growth of natural health products* as more exploration of the Amazon River basin and other regions increases.

Earnings of pharmaceutical firms may fall as more persons are treated with natural health substances. My guess is that as physicians begin to use natural health treatments they will be delighted by the efficacy and safety of these therapies.

The era of pharmaceutical dominance of the health care market has started to diminish. Many concerned patients are trying to opt out of the use of drugs and are pursuing natural treatments for their health problems. These people are searching for physicians who can guide them in use of natural substances. My hope is that this book will help bridge the gap for both groups.

The June 2000 Journal of the American Medical Association published an article, which documented that *the fourth leading cause of death is disease caused by medical treatment!*

Many of these deaths relate to adverse reactions from drugs. The multiple adverse reactions from the many available pharmaceutical agents are very difficult to remember and this becomes compounded when the patient is taking 6- 15 medicines *all of which have new untoward reactions with each other.*

Fortunately there are natural treatments for all diseases that are much easier for the body to cope with and which do not have nearly as many dangerous side effects. That's what this book is all about. *Governmental expenses for health care will fall* substantially and these funds can be returned to the taxpayers or placed into other programs.

About The Food We Eat

Just when everything seems hopeless for the family farmer because of low commodity prices an important horticultural breakthrough has occurred. Plants have tiny openings in their leaves called *stomata*. These stomata are used to *inhale* carbon dioxide and *exhale* oxygen and water.

Dr. T.C. Singh, Head of the Department of Botany at the Annamali University in India discovered that when he played music to the plants at 6 AM for 30 minutes daily, within two weeks the number of stomata on the plant leaf had increased by 66%. Not only were the numbers of stomata increased but also the plants exhibited above average growth and rates of growth. Dr. Singh's conclusion was that he had been able to prove *that harmonic sound waves affect the growth, flowering, fruiting and seed-yields of many plants.*

Dan Carlson developed a burning desire to help alleviate the world's hunger when he saw people starving to death overseas during a severe drought. When he returned to the United States he enrolled in the Experimental College at the University of Minnesota. His research was able to reveal some sound frequencies, which caused plant stomata to open. A music teacher named Michael Holtz, while helping him make an audiotape of these frequencies, *advised him that these frequencies were nearly identical to the frequencies and harmonics of bird sounds at the beginning of the day.*

Mr. Carlson then decided to confirm that these sound harmonics would stimulate plant growth. He bought a Purple Passion vine and began playing harmonics similar to bird music, while simultaneously applying nutrient to the leaves with a cotton swab. Over a 3 month period, the plant had grown to 150 feet. By the end of one year, the plant was 600 feet long. The normal maximum size of this plant is only 24 inches.

The next year he sold starts from his plant. Excited buyers began to call him, telling him the plants had rapidly grown to 30 to 50 feet. Carlson contacted the *Guinness Book of Records* and after investigation, they accepted his 600 foot long Purple Passion vine as the world record holder. This plant eventually reached 1,200 feet in length. The vine not only grew large but it blossomed more frequently than usual. Successive generations of the plant had apparently achieved favorable genetic changes as the seeds produced new generations that were larger and more fruitful than their parents.

A farmer named Ron Johnson knew about Carlson's research and constructed some boxes eight feet by 16 feet and filled them with sawdust and sand. He used special bacteria (possibly SBO) from France in the soil and daily played Carlson's bird-like sounds. Once each week he sprayed the leaves with foliar solution. His tomato plants, which were seven inches apart, produced 25 to 30 blossoms and yielded 16 pounds of fruit per plant. Some tomatoes weighed one and a half pounds. Each box produced one thousand pounds of tomatoes.

Another box of the same size planted with 200 strawberry plants produced two hundred quarts of tasty, nutritious strawberries. There was no rain for 6 weeks, the temperature was over 100 degrees F. daily and this was poor soil. This system needs very little watering, no plowing and no cultivating, with very little weeding. A box could produce 800 cantaloupes and enough beans to feed a family of four for one year.

An apple farmer accustomed to getting 210 bushels per acre is now getting 450 bushels an acre. Ninety percent of these apples are "packable". (Good enough to display.) This is compared to 50% previously.

Mr. Carlson states that if he sprays nutrient on any fruit tree at petal tight stage and bouquet bloom stage he gets a four percent set instead of the usual one and a half percent set. Probably the most important part of this new style of farming is that the apples have a 400% increase in copper, 1,750% increase in zinc, 300% increase in chromium and 126% increase in potassium. The apples are two sizes larger, much better tasting and much more nutritious. Black walnuts are as large as oranges, corn plants are 16 feet high and potatoes are the size of 1 liter bottles.

Mr. Carlson's findings have the potential to save the small farmer and give the public far better food.

What we eat plays a vital role in our health. My hope is that access to more nutritious produce will improve health as more people grow their own organic produce on that little plot of land in the back yard and have better, safer and more nutritious food

More information can be obtained from Bio/Tech News P.O.Box 30568 Parkrose Center, Portland, OR 97294. Request their special report *Super Sonic.* Contact Josef's Storhaus to purchase Sonic Bloom or to request The Home and Garden Kit, which includes the cassette tape. 800-535-3587.

A Final Note

We intend to build *Natural Health Team* into a unique company in partnership with those we serve. We have selected treatments that all appear to have great merit. However, it is vital to us that we receive feedback by email, fax or letter from you about the results of using the products we recommend. This feedback will enable us to identify and eliminate any product that fails to provide positive results.

May God bless you with better health.

Dr James A Howenstine- *Natural Health Team*

Website: www.naturalhealthteam.com

Address: 7333 NW 54th St. Miami, FL 33166

Email: doctorjim@naturalhealthteam.com

Products and this book can be purchased by calling 800-416-2806.

Acknowledgements

This book is not based on my work alone. My 34 years experience of caring for patients in office and hospitals, has been combined with ideas and concepts obtain from the research and study of my colleagues..

I am very grateful to Dr. David Williams for the many exciting insights he has provided in his *Alternatives*. Dr. Julian Whitaker in his *Health and Healing* has added many valuable ideas about how natural health therapy can effectively replace pharmaceuticals in caring for a wide variety of problems.

Much valuable information about immunizations found in Chapter 29 was obtained from Dr. Ralph Rowen's brochure "Your First Consultation with Dr. Rowen".

Many cutting edge insights into new natural therapies have been gleaned from *Health Sciences Institute*. I have been helped by the insights of Dr. John McDougall's *To Your Health*. *Bio/Tech News* has provided information about several wonderful new healing substances as well as the data about growing better food by playing audiotapes similar to bird harmonics.

The scholarly scientific approach of William I. Fischer's book, *How To Fight Cancer and Win* has been very helpful. I am particularly grateful for Dr. Joanna Budwig's program for treating cancer with flax oil and cottage cheese.

Eustace Mullin's book, *Murder By Injection,* was of great value for the historical information obtained about fluoridation, immunization and the contamination of our food supply. I am grateful to Dr. Robert Atkins for the information about taurine and the case report of the comatose girl following root canal surgery.

Several of the food ideas from Dr. Stephen Sinatra's *Health Report* have been incorporated into the book as well as his ideas about diastolic heart failure. Invaluable information about the cause and cure of Type 2 diabetes was obtained from Thomas Smith's book *Insulin: Our Silent Killer*. The information about irradiation of food and the problems of meat were obtained from the October, 2001 *Townsend Letter for Doctors and Patients*.

Much of the material about mercury toxicity from dental amalgams was found in Gary Null's *Living Natural*.

The data about essential oils came from BioTech News and the December 2001 issue of the Townsend Letters for Doctors and Patients.

I must also thank Dr. Jack Dawkins, Doug Del Tondo, and Colin Benner have reviewed this book and contributed worthwhile suggestions.

Lastly and most important this book never would have become a reality without the encouragement that my friend Clinton Cruickshank gave me to pursue my dreams about the importance of natural health care.

While I thank each of the above, I am solely responsible for the contents, views and opinions expressed in this book.

An attempt has been made to place important information in each chapter that will be of value to you, your family and your friends.

Appendix "A"

How To Use This Table

How to preventing drug-induced nutrient deficiencies

You can determine any nutrient deficiencies that may be present in your body from taking medications by using this reference guide. Nutrient depletion can be a serious problem and can cause cardiac disorders, hearing loss, memory loss, a lowered immune response, depression, fatigue, muscle weakness, anemia, hair loss and other complications.

We encourage you to refer to this chart.

1. Locate medications you take and note any nutrient depletion associated with them.

2. Consult the recommended supplement guidelines.

3. If a nutrient is depleted by two or more different medications, add together the recommended supplement amounts for each drug, but do not exceed the *maximum* recommended dosage amount for each nutrient.

4. Check the dosages for nutrients provided by any nutritional supplements you may *already* take.

5. Supplement your regimen as necessary with additional nutrients

Our special thanks for *HEALTH SCIENCES INSTITUTE* for permission to use this most valuable chart.

This chart *Preventing Drug-Induced Nutrient Deficiences* was obtained from the Drug-Induced Nutrient Depletion Handbook by Ross Pelton, James B Lavalle, Ernest B. Hawkins and Donald L. Krinsky (Hudson, OH: Lexi-Comp, 1999)

Type of Drug	Names/ brands	Nutrients Depleted	Deficiency symptoms and risk factors	Recommended supplemental dosage	Max. recomm. amount from all sources
cid-blocking ugs - used for cers, digestion, ERD					
-2 Agonists	Pepcid (famatodine) Tagamet (cimetidine) Zantac (tranitidine)	Vitamin B-12	Anemia, fatigue, increased risk of heart disease	100-1000mg.	1,000-2,000 mcg. Rx only
		Folic Acid	Anymia,birth defects,cervical dysplasia,increased riskof heart disease	800mcg.	> 1-2 mg. Rx only
		Vitamin D	Osteoporosis, muscle weakness, hearing loss	400 IU	400 IU>800 IU linked with fibrosis
		Calcium	Osteoporosis, muscle weakness, irregularities	500-1000 mg.	1,000 -1,500 mg.
		Iron	Anemia, fatigue,hair loss, brittle nails	10-50 mg. from calcium	>50mg.may cause constipation
		Zinc	Lowered immunity, loss of sense of smell and taste, slow wound healing	50mg	75 mg., excess depletes copper
oton Pump hibitors	Prevacid (lansoprazole) Prilosec (omeprasole)	Vitamin B-12	Anemia, fatigue, increased risk of heart disease	100-1,000mcg.	1,000-2,000 mcg. - Rx only
olesterol- wering drugs					

Cholesterol- lowering drugs				

HMG-CoA reductase inhibitors	Bayacol (cerivastatin) Lescol (fluvastatin) Lipitor (atorvastatin) Mevacor (lovastatin) Zocor (simvastatin)	Co enzyme Q-10	Low energy, depressed immune function, high blood pressure, congestive heart failure	30-100 mg.	600 mg. Test Serum Co-Q-10 level to verify absorption
Bile-acid sequestrants	Questran (cholestyramine) Colestid (colestipol)	Vitamin A	Night blindness, skin disorders increased risk of cancers	10,000 IU	25,000 IU. Take higher amounts for short periods only
		Beta-carotene	Night bliness, skin disorders increased risk of cancers	10,000 IU	10-25,000 IU Take higher amounts for shor periods only
		Vitamin B-12	Anemia, fatigue, increased risk of heart disease	100-1,000 mcg.	1,000-2,000 mcg - Rx only
		Vitamin D	See Vitamin D above		
		Vitamin E	Dry skin, brittle nails, PMS, eczema, psoriasis, benign prostatic hyperplasia	400 IU	800 IU
		Vitamin K	Abnormal blood clotting (easy bleeding or bruising) osteoporosis	I mg.	10 mg. Rx only for 1 week

		Folic acid	See Folic Acid above		
		Iron	See Iron above		
ntidepressents					
ricyhclic ntidepressants	Adapin (doxepin) Elavil (amitriptyline) Tofranil (imipramine)	Coenzyme Q-10	Lower energy, depressed immune function, high blood pressure, congestive heart failure	30-100 mg.	600 mg., Test serum Co-Q-112 level to verify verify absorption
ntidiabetic drugs					
olfonylureas	Dymelor (acetohexaminde) Micronase (glyburide) Tolinase (tolazamide)	Coenzyme Q-10	Low energy, drepressed immune function, high blood pressure congestive heart failure	30-100 mg.	600 mg., Test serum Co-Q-10 level to verify absorbtion
iguanides ides	Glucophage (metformin)	Vitamin B-12	See above		
ntihypertensives (used to lower blood pressure)					
asodilators ilators	Apresoline (hydralazine)	Vitamin B-6	Anemia, fatigue, depression, increased risk of heart disease	50 mg.	150 mg.
		Coenzyme Q-10	See above		
oop Diuretics	Bumex (bumetanide	Vitamin B-1	Depression, memory loss, muscle weakness	50 mg.	100 mg.
	Edecrin (ethacrynic acid) Lasix (furosemide)	Vitamin B-6	See above		
		Vitamin C	Lowered immune response, poor wound healing	1,000mg.	10,000 mg. or to bowel tolerance which varies

		Magnesium	Cardiovascular irregularities, asthmaas, osteoporosis, Muscle cramps	250-500 mg.	500-800 mg.ma cause loose stoo
		Calcium	Osteoporosis, cardiac irregularies	5,00-1,000mg.	1,000-1,500 mg
		Potassium	Irregular heartbeat, muscle weakness, fatigue	99-198 mg.	198-297 mg. Higher dosage b Rx
		Zinc	Lowered immunity, loss of sense of smell and taste,slow wound healing	50 mg.	75 mg.- excess depletes copper
Thiazide diuretics	Aquatensen (methyclothiazide)	Coenzyme Q10	Coenzyme Q10 above		
	Lozol (indapamide)	Magnesium	See Magnesium above		
	Zaroxolyn (metalozone)	Zinc	See Zinc above		
Potassium sparing diuretics	Dyrenium (triamterene)	Folic Acid	See Folic Acid below		
		Calcium	See Calcium above		
		Zinc	See Zinc above		

eta-blockers	Biocadren (timolol) Cartrol (carteolol) Inderal (propranolol) Lopressor (metoprolol) Normodyne (labetalol Sectral (acebutolol) Tenormin (tenolol) Kerlone (betaxolol) Viskin (pindolol)	Coenzyme Q-10	Low energy, depressed immune function, high blood pressure, congestive heart failure.	30-50mg.	600 mg. Test serum Co-Q-10 level to verify absorption
Anti-inflammatories					
Salicylates	Aspirin	Vitamin C	See Vitamin C above		
		Folic Acid	See Folic acid below		
		Iron	See Iron above		
		Potassium	See Potassium above		
NSAIDS	Advil, Aleve, Dolobid, Feldene, Indocene, Lodine, Naprosyn, Orudis, Relafen, Voltaren	Folic Acid	Anemia, birth defects, cervical displasia, increased risk of heart disease	600 mcg.	> 1-2 mg.Rx only
Corticosteroids	Betamethasone, Budesonide, Cortisone, Dexamasone, Hydrocortisone, Methylprednisolone	Vitamin C	See Vitamin C above		
		Vitamin D	See Vitamin D above		
		Folic Acid	See Folic Acid above		

		Calicium	See Calcium above		
		Magnesium	See Magnesium above		
		Potassium	See Potassium above		
	Prednisone	Selinium	Lowered immune response, increased risk of cancer, reduced antioxidantprotection	100 mcg.	200 mcg.
	Predisolone	Zinc	See Zinc above		
Oral Contraceptives	Estrastep	Vitamin B-2	Skin disorders	50 mg.	100 mg.
	Norinyl, Ortho-Novem,	Vitamin B-6	Anemia, fatigue, depression, increased risk of heart disease	50 mg.	150 mg.
	Tripasil and others	Vitamin B-12	Anemia, fatigue, increased risk of heart disease	100-1,000 mcg.	1,000-2,000 mcg Rx only
		Folic Acid	Anemia, birth defects, cervical dysplasia, increased risk of heart diseases	800 mcg.	>1-2 mg. Rx only
		Vitamin C	Lowered immune response, poor wound healing	1,000 mg.	10,000 mg. or to bowel tolerance which varies
		Magnesium	See Magnisium above		
		Zinc	Lowered immunity, loss of sense of smell and taste, slow wound healing		75mg. excess depletes copper

rmone lacement rapy	Evista (raloxifine), Prempro, Premarin, Estratab and others	Vitamin B-2	See Vitamin B-2 above		
		Vitamin B-6	See Vitamin B-6 above		
		Vitamin B-12	See Viitamin B-12 above		
		Folic Acid	See Folic Avid above		
		Vitamin C	See Vitamin C above		
		Magnesium	See Magnesium above		
		Zinc	See Zinc above		
anquilizers					
nothyazines	Ormazine	Vitamin B-2	Skin disorders	50 mg.	100 mg.
	Thorazine (chlorpromazine)	Coenzyme Q-10	Low energy, depressed immune function, high blood pressure, congestive heart failure	30-100 mg.	600 mg. Test serum Co-Q10 to verify absorbtion
	Mellaril (thioridazine)				
	Prolixin (fluphenazine)				
tyrophenones	Haldol (haloperidol)	Coenzyme Q-10	Low energy, depressed immune function, high blood pressure, congestive heart failure	30-100 mg.	600 mg. Test serum Co-Q10 to verify absorption

ALPHABETICAL LIST OF DISEASES IN BOOK

I

VITILIGO 175
VOMITING 80

Y

YERSINIA 117

– NOTES –

– NOTES –

– NOTES –

– NOTES –

– NOTES –

– NOTES –

Made in the USA